Acknowledgements

Though Jason and I are the creators of the Eat Well Bible, we could not have done it without the support and assistance from the whole team. We would, in particular, like to acknowledge and thank Lee Jones and Jefferson Gler for the photography, design, creativity and dedication in making the first Eat Well Bible a reality.

Jason would like thank Gemma Hill for the support and encouragement in creating and refining these recipes, for the belief in the project and the patience shown during the many late nights and early mornings spent writing.

Personally, I would like to thank every member of TEAM Boot Camp and the hundreds of campers that make Heydour House an amazing working (and living!) environment. I am immensely proud of everything we do at TEAM and look forward to what promises to be an amazing future.

Finally, I would like to thank the single biggest reason I feel alive each day, my greatest ally and the future Mrs. Williams, Paula. She deserves permanent and very public recognition for constantly greasing the wheels and creating the perfect environment for people to change.

About TEAM Bootcamp

Launched in August 2013 by Paula Howell & Craig Williams, TEAM Bootcamp quickly established a reputation for hard, no compromise military style training on the outside and soft, caring support on the inside. Based in Heydour House in Lincolnshire, TEAM helps hundreds of people Think, Eat and Move differently in pursuit of rapidly improved fitness and fat loss

If you want to rapidly boost fitness and scorch calories in a relaxing and nurturing environment, visit team-bootcamp.com or Like us on Facebook at www.facebook.com/TeamBootcamp3d

----

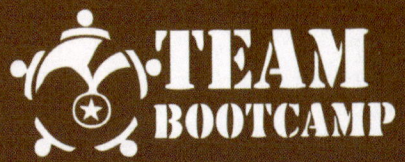

Section 1 - Health & nutrition tips for health and weight management

Section 2 - Introduction to Paleo nutrition

Chapter 1 - Breakfast
Chapter 2 - Snacks
Chapter 3 - Lamb
Chapter 4 - Beef
Chapter 5 - Seafood
Chapter 6 - Chicken
Chapter 7 - Pork
Chapter 8 - Vegetarian
Chapter 9 - Soups
Chapter 10 - Sauces

Section 3 - Resources

Contents

Introduction..3
But First a Little about Me..3
Create a Deep Rooted Desire..10
The V2W Principle.. 10
Enabling Change..11
Solid Foundations..14
Triggers to Unhealthy Eating...16
Sleep Yourself Thin...18
Sleep to Grow..19
Food is Fuel...21
Food is Information...21
Discipline Your Insulin..22
Balanced Meals...23
Carbohydrates..24
Protein...24
Fats..25
Water...26
Crash Prevention...27
Make Smart Choices Easy...28
Tackle Sabotage...28
Preparation is Key...29
Make It a Habit..30

SECTION 1 - INTRODUCTION

If you are reading this, then you may have participated in my nutrition seminars or workshops or have spoken to someone that has. Whichever it is, you have obviously made a conscious decision to change your image and get your health in shape.

The bad news: despite what many fad diets will have you believe, getting your weight in check can be quite a challenge. It will take some real, sustained effort and determination. The good news: this book contains all the information you need to get your lifelong journey off to a great start.

But First a Little about Me

Paula, the TEAM and I coach hundreds to think, eat and move better at TEAM Boot Camp by infusing the lessons and strategies I developed through my own health and weight loss journey, but what about life before TEAM?

As a personal trainer, celebrity bootcamp instructor and former royal marine, you probably think I naturally have a great image. The truth is that I have been through the mill a little with regards to weight.

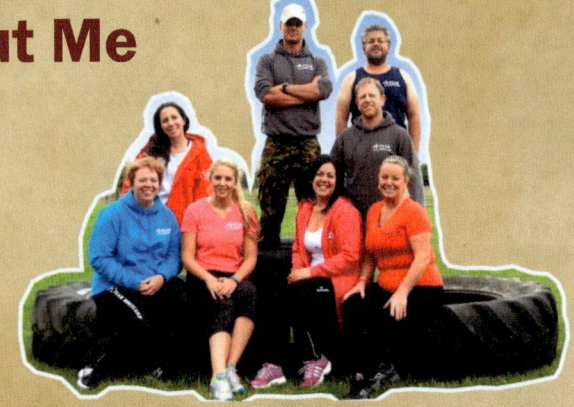

TEAM BOOTCAMP

I understand the physical and emotional highs and lows with regards to carrying excess weight and having poor eating habits all too well. As a young marine, I picked up the nickname 'Pie Shop' and was put on a calorie-controlled diet during training because of my 'rotund' appearance. That's a bit of a kick in the obvious when you are in the top 0.1% of the fittest young men in the world.

Training for the Royal Marines is some of the most arduous training in the world. It lasts 32 weeks and involves yomping, crawling and running mile after mile and jumping, climbing and swimming your way to an elite level of fitness. Few people ever experience that intensity of the training, and I did it all when I was supposedly in my prime, So why was I still fat? Why was I embarrassed when I stood there in my budgie smugglers next to 45 others with the bodies of Adonis while I sported love handles and man boobs?

> " Why, if I reportedly scorched 5,500 calories on an easy day in training, was I making myself sick in an effort to ditch the blubber, and why was I desperately seeking answers in one fad diet after the next? "

Finding the answer was a long journey of study, trial and error and eventual discovery, but the good news is that I got there. The better news is that I can help you, and the BEST news is the foundations to a fitter healthier you. The essence of my journey from self-conscious, lardy marine to celebrity personal trainer, bootcamp instructor and wellness coach is contained here in this section of the Eat Well Bible. The best news is that because you are reading this, you have already taken the hardest step.

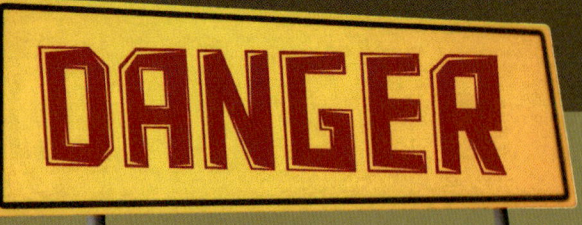

DANGER: Please remember that you will have to make some sacrifices to really achieve what you desire and what you have been searching for throughout the years. You are always in danger of not achieving lifelong results because you put things off and fail to do what's necessary to get what you want. Simply reading the book or even attending one of the TEAM Boot Camp weight loss camps is not enough. You have to put the steps into practice. Don't wait until tomorrow because tomorrow never comes. Work hard today and be proud tomorrow!

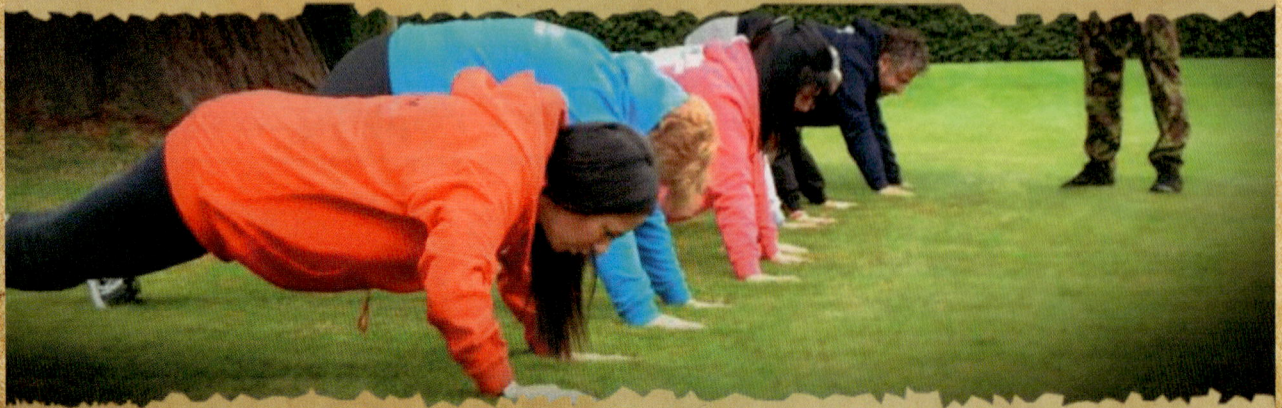

Create a Deep-rooted Desire

With the right motivation, you can achieve anything you set your mind to. Your first step in achieving anything must be establishing your motivation. To help you, I would like to share a principle that I created while coaching young men preparing to join the elite military forces.

Now, we know you have no interest in kicking in doors or abseiling through windows to rescue hostages, but this principle can be just as powerful in your pursuit of an improved image or increased health. It can help you create the motivation and desire to get going, slowly building the momentum when creating habits that will last you for forever.

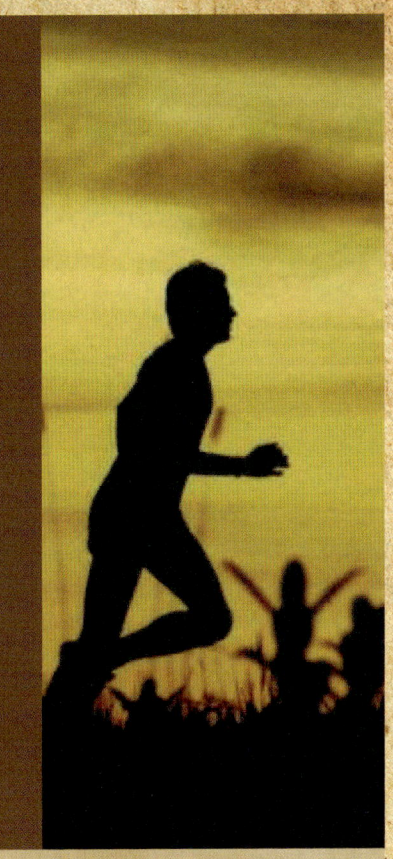

The V2W Principle

The three components of the V2W Principle are powerful tools in their own right, but when they are combined, their effectiveness knows no bounds. V2W stands for Visualise, What, Why and is explained in more depth below.

V - VISUALISE

Visualisation is an age-old technique for creating motivation, but it's one that many see as a little too fairy-like for them. However, I am a great advocate of the fact that if the mind can conceive it, the body can achieve it. If your internal dialogue is spattered with — I can't...,""I could never...," or "I won't be able to...,"then you're doomed. You're making a very common mistake that sabotages many people's progress every day. The minute we say — I can't," the mind stops looking for options, opportunities and answers. It acts like a shutoff valve to being positive and successful.

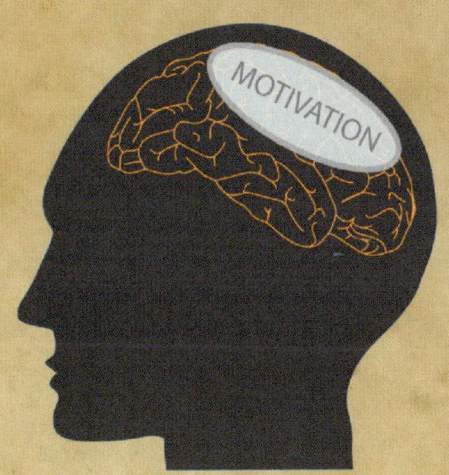

Visualise the fitter, faster or leaner you in the future. Imagine how your clothes will look and feel and how proud you will be as people comment on your slimmer hips and slender thighs.

W - WHAT

Ask yourself WHAT you will gain from eating cleaner and healthier. What are the benefits that matter to you? What is it that will propel you on when all you want to do is jump off the wagon and smash the backside out a tub of Ben & Jerry's? It's the end results or the final outcomes that will motivate you, and we need to hardwire our thoughts to focus on whatever it is now so our mind is anchored to them when things get tough.

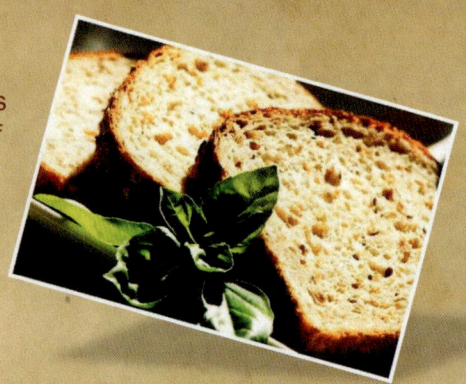

W - WHY

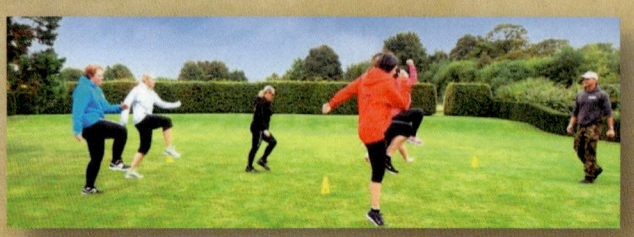

Listing the reasons WHY you want to manage your weight or improve your fitness can be very powerful. Constant reminders help you stay in the produce aisle and out of the bakery or chocolate section of the supermarket. Take a few seconds to sit without interruption and list the reasons why you're reading this now.

Finally, I wish you the very best of luck, though wishing you luck suggests that you are leaving something to chance! To be honest, you are about to stack the odds in your favour with simple, no BS tips, techniques and advice to take control of your eating and recruiting your body's natural functions as an ally in your battle against poor food choices.

Craig Williams, formerly 'Pie Shop,' and three-time world pork pie eating champ, 95-97, 99 (I was on operations in 98!)

Enabling Change

You will never change anything if you continue to do the same things, and doing the same thing over and over and expecting a different result is insane. So some things are simply going to have to change. At first glance, changing and forming new habits seem hard, but actually, it's easy. We form new habits every day. We have a particular morning routine. We shop in a certain way and even get dressed habitually. So they're easy to form; we just need to be a little more conscious of them. The tough part is forming good habits that sadly go against what is considered the norm.

It's human nature to always take the path of least resistance, and eating poorly is easy. It's often cheaper, quicker and, in some respects, tastier, but the Eat Well Bible hopes to redefine your idea of 'normal.'

At TEAM Boot Camp, we prescribe a paleo dietary plan, also known as the caveman or primal diet, which, if you don't know, reflects how our palaeolithic ancestors would have eaten pre-farming and before we started processing food. You will find an explanation of paleo in Section 2 of this book, and for those that would like a deeper understanding, I recommend reading Robb Wolf or Loren Cordain, authors of *The Paleo Solution* and *The Paleo Diet*, respectively. In this section, we will teach you genuine weight loss principles to help you improve the WAY you eat, not what you eat.

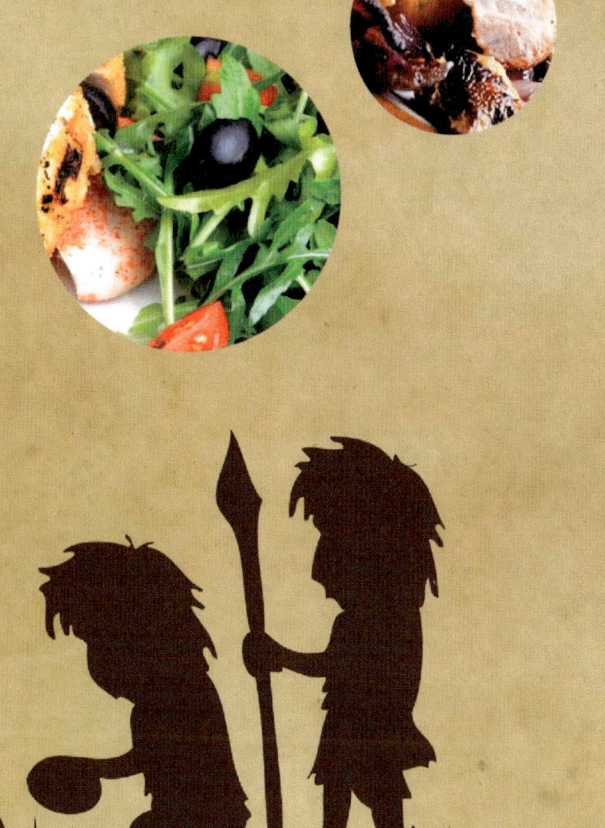

Remember : don't try to change everything all at once! Start with some of the big hitters. For example, when I train, I naturally and automatically want to eat cleaner. So creating the habit to train most days has made eating cleaner a by-product. These are known as keystone habits; take a few minutes to consider what some of your keystone habits are.

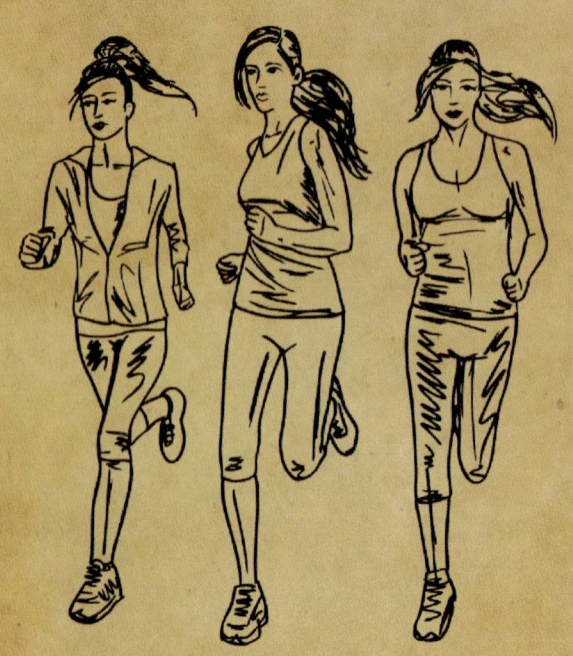

Solid Foundations

In order to succeed in your health and fitness goals, you are going to require three vital ingredients, sound nutrition, effective fitness training and sufficient rest. They seem obvious, but actually, many people fail in their quest because they forget the words *sound*, *effective* and *sufficient*. Each component must be layered, starting with a solid foundation of sound nutrition.

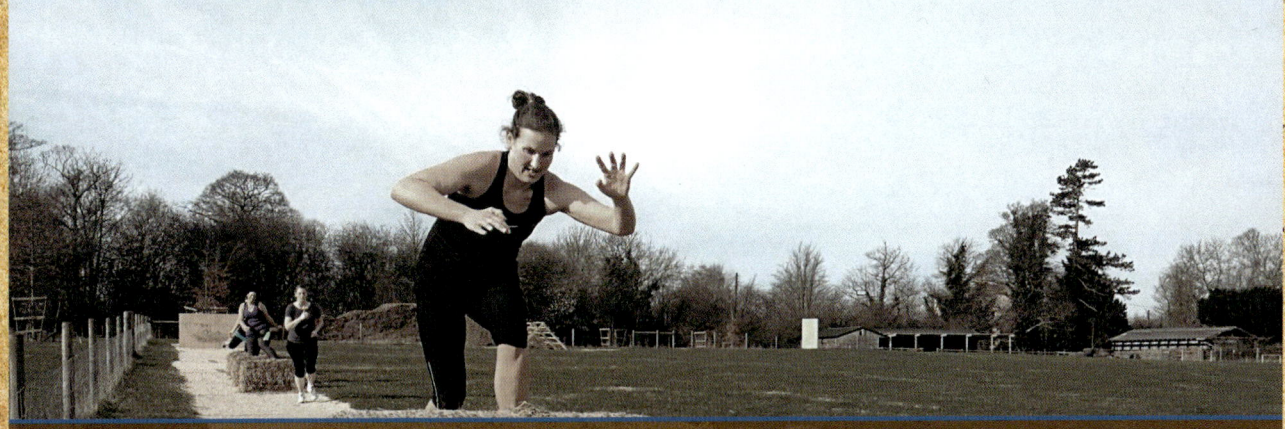

In conjunction with good, clean eating, exercise will aid in your weight management, fitness and health, but beware that many people see exercise as the answer and fail to realise that reaching your goals really is 80% eating and only 20% exercise.

Stop looking for the answer in the gym or in exercise.

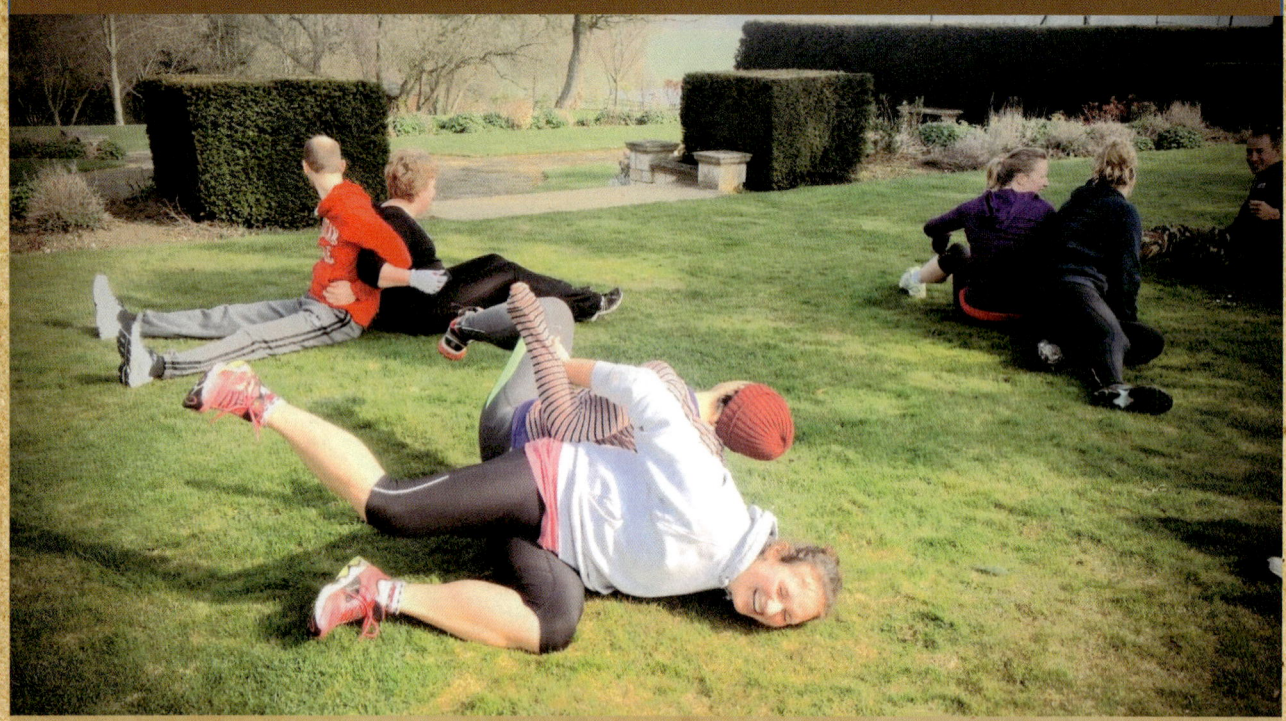

You will never out-train poor nutrition. Exercise certainly forms some of the answer to your weight loss journey, but actually, too much exercise can have a negative effect, especially if your training is ineffective.

TRIGGERS TO UNHEALTHY EATING

In my experience, there is rarely an occasion when a person makes a poor food choice where there hasn't been a 'trigger' of some form. An example is the time when you've had a terrible day at work, and the last thing you want to do now that you're home is cook dinner. You grab the dog-eared takeaway menu and order the usual. You deserve a night off, right?

Identifying your own individual triggers is a major step in achieving your weight management goals. Learning to recognise the emotions, occasions or events that trigger unhealthy eating will immediately give you the upper hand.

During my time in the Marines, I learnt to identify combat indicators. It was the only weapon we had against an unidentifiable enemy employing terror tactics rather than engaging in more traditional fighting. Combat indicators are the 'presence of the abnormal,' or 'absence of the normal,' and every soldier is taught to recognise the often slightest sign that trouble is brewing. Many lives are saved when the signs that something isn't quite right are noticed. It could be anything from displaced soil, indicating a buried explosive device, or an absence of civilians in a normally thriving marketplace, which could indicate the threat of a suicide bomber.

Action Points

Step one

Allocate a little time to consider your triggers to unhealthy eating. It is also helpful to catch yourself during your unhealthy eating periods to consider the situation, emotions or events that led to poor choices.

Step two

Armed with your list of unhealthy eating triggers, now consider all the ways to combat these triggers.

SLEEP YOURSELF THIN

Sounds too easy, right? You can make things significantly easier for yourself by understanding the body's natural reaction to crave sugary foods during the summer when days are long and the nights are short. As cavemen, we evolved to crave food during the summer season when fruits, berries, honey and other natural sources of simple sugars were plentiful in order to fatten up for the cold, harsh winter months. The issue comes in modern times with the fact that our bodies are fooled into believing we are in a constant state of summer or a constant state of 'getting fat for winter.' The light bulb allows us to treat night as day, unlike our ancestors, who would have been forced to wrap up for the night and sleep until dawn.

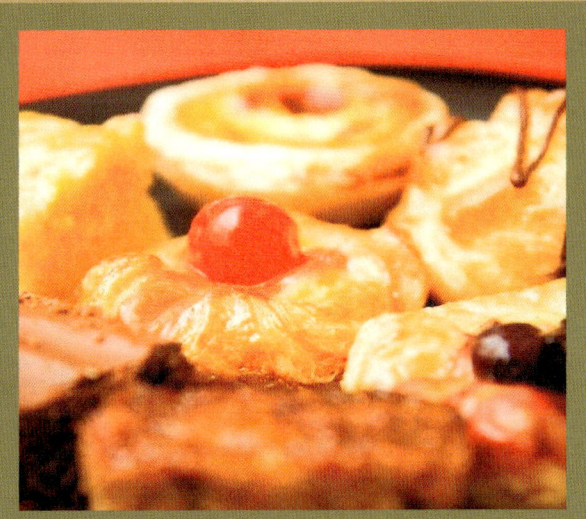

In order to use sleep and long nights to our advantage, we must aim for about 8-9 hours of sleep per night. That sounds like a lot, but again, once we make better, more consistent and effective sleep habitual, you soon develop the sleeping ability of a dormouse.

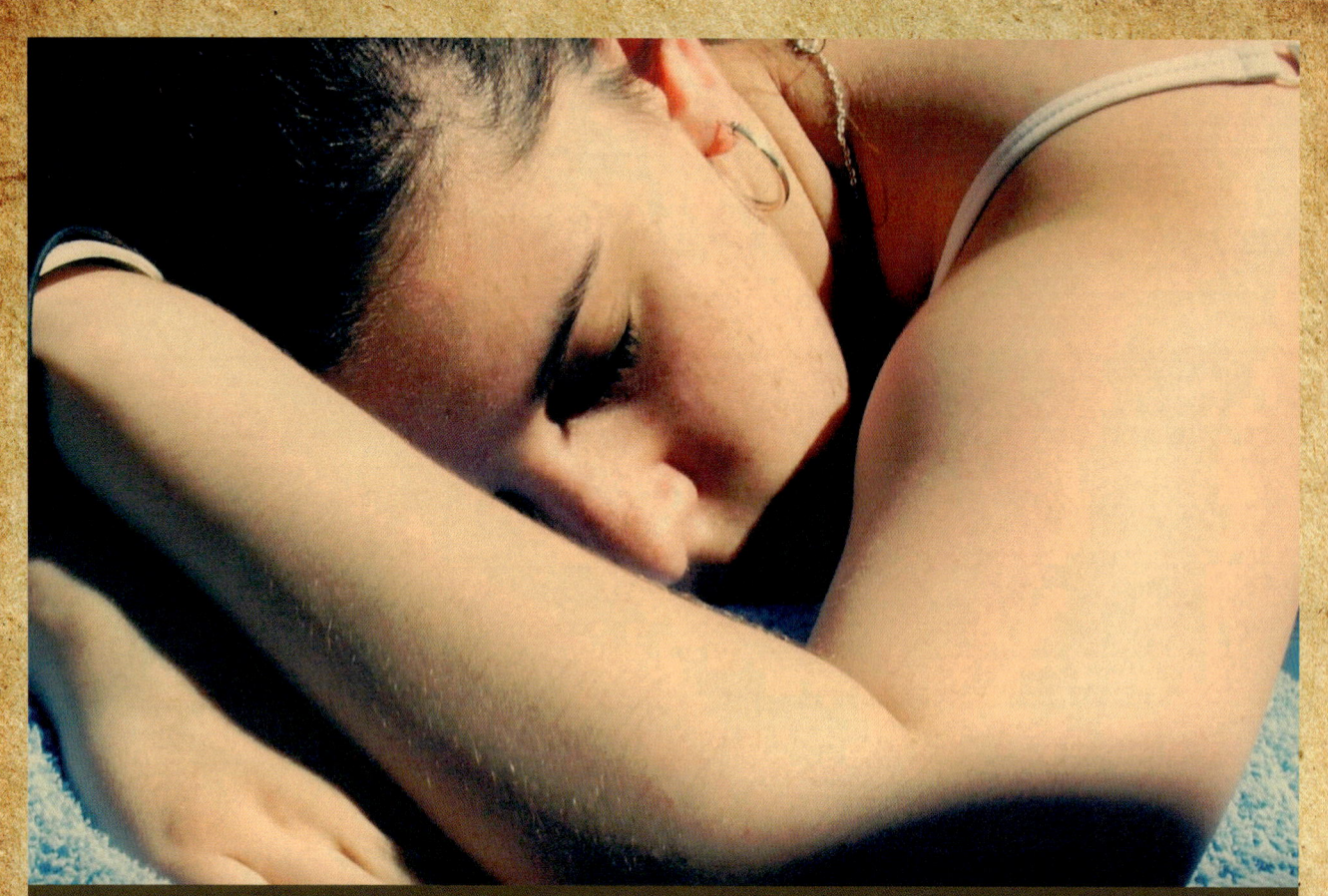

Additional benefits of sleeping longer include a reduction in the nasty bacteria that develop in the gut throughout the day and a reduction in cortisol levels (responsible for the storage of fat, particularly around the stomach and waist), which counteract the fat-burning hormone testosterone. You may feel sceptical about this, and you are right to feel that way. So I suggest that you try it or at least be more aware of what's happening in your body the next time you fail to get a good night's sleep. Mild effects include an increased desire for fast food, especially sugary, fatty and salty foods, and extreme effects can include gut irritation and ache due to the build-up of bacteria and their waste products in the gut.

Here are a few tips for getting the optimum amount of rest:

- ❖ **Black out** - Even the smallest amount of light can cause the receptors in the skin to trigger the sugar craving signals telling us to get fat in preparation for winter.
- ❖ **Avoid alcohol** - Though you may find it easier to drift off to sleep, alcohol-induced sleep is often disrupted, leaving you feeling fatigued and unrested.
- ❖ **Avoid stimulants** - Caffeine and other stimulants can prevent you from getting to sleep and leave you pacing the bedroom for hours. Reduce your stimulant intake after midday.

It is hard for many people to accept that the body does not get fitter, faster and leaner in the gym. It is during rest that the body repairs and recovers that little bit stronger and fitter in adaptation to the stresses we placed on it through exercise. View sleeping more as healing rather than just sleep. It helps you to keep the importance of good-quality sleep in perspective.

The body repairs itself fully during the deep REM stage of sleep. Typically, this takes approximately 4 hours. Aim for 2 cycles of REM sleep per night to truly maximise your gains.

Food is Fuel

With foods scientifically engineered to excite every taste receptor in our mouths, it is hard sometimes to remember that food is actually just two things: fuel and information. This paragraph deals with the fuel aspect. In simple terms, every food has a determined amount of energy that will be absorbed by the body. If you eat more than you use, the body will convert a high percentage of the excess energy to fat to be stored in our fuel tanks: the hips, thighs, love handles and bingo wings!

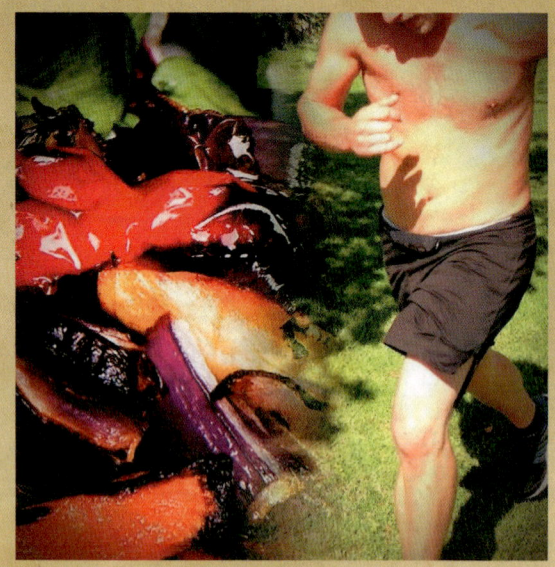

Food is Information

The body also uses food as information to control its basic functions, such as hormonal messages to get more sugar or say, ―Stop eating― I am full." Improving your knowledge of the food groups, including knowing what each do and what information they provide, can significantly contribute to your ability to cope with and overcome cravings and prevent you from dropping well into the crash zone.

The great news is that all the recipes and the principles in this book will help feed the body with the right information, even without you knowing it.

DISCIPLINE YOUR INSULIN

Insulin plays a huge part in the storage of fat, the use of energy in the body and the cravings for naff food. Learning to prevent erratic peaks and drops in your blood sugar levels and insulin can make weight loss and healthy living easier. I suggest reading *The Blood Sugar Solution* by Mark Hyman to learn all about the effects of food and the messages different ingredients send.

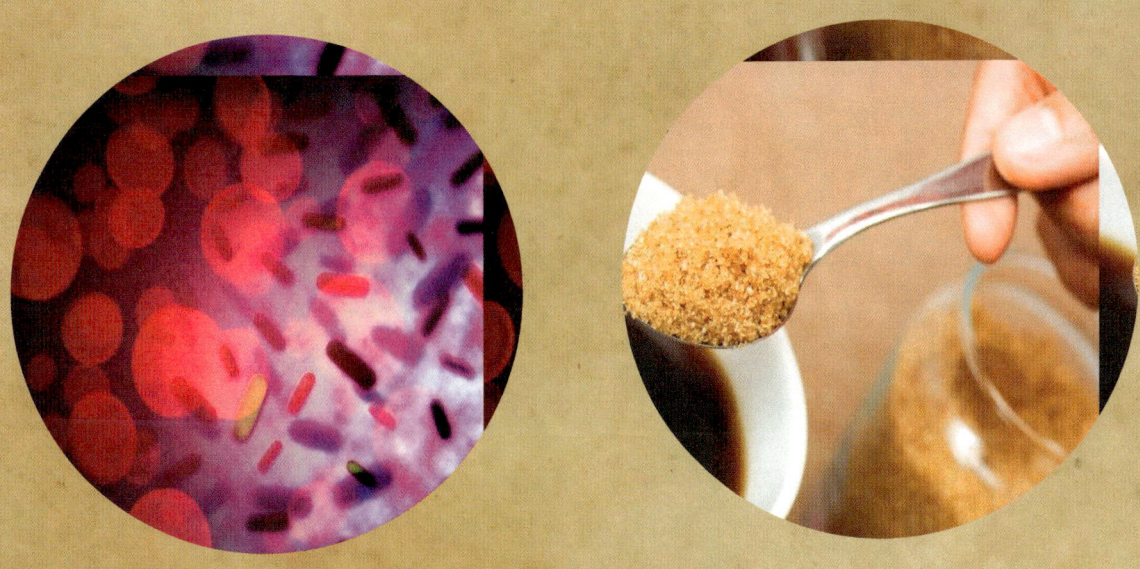

BALANCED MEALS

Though many of our basic processes slow at night, the body is constantly performing all the functions that keep us fit and healthy. These processes require nutrients that we obtain from food. Therefore, we need to ensure that the body has a constant supply of every food group throughout the day.

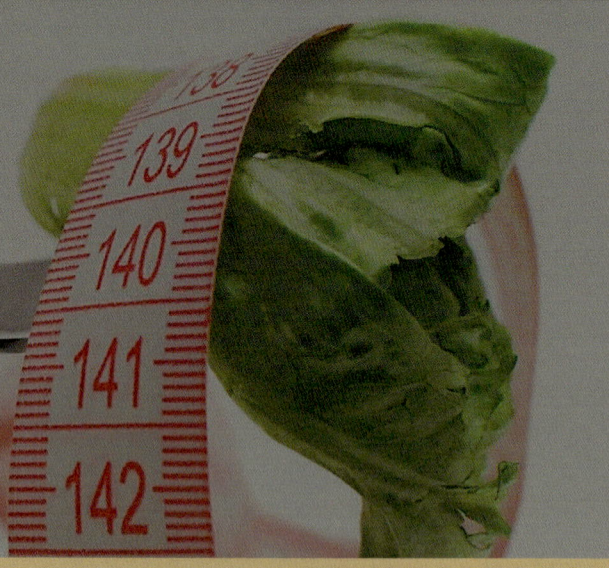

Over the next few weeks, you will develop a number of default meals containing an almost optimal amount of protein, fats and carbohydrates for your body's requirements. Consuming balanced meals will ensure that you provide your body with everything it needs each time you eat. Benefits of eating in this manner are prevention of potential starvation periods, a boost in nutrient intake, slowing of the digestion process as well as a regulation of the fat storage hormone, insulin.

Eating in a balanced manner is a little tough at first purely because we have been conditioned to eat carb-focused breakfasts, snacks and lunches and only make a concerted effort to include protein for dinner.

What follows is an overview of the basic food groups and the functions they have in the body. If we know and understand what the food groups are, we can ensure that we always have balanced meals.

Carbohydrates

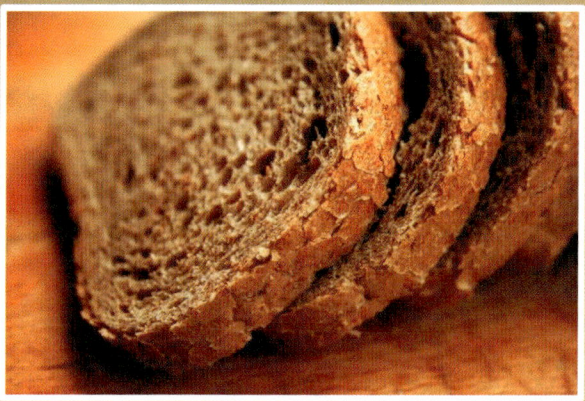

What they do - Provide energy and control the release of insulin.

Your approximate amount - Aim for 2 fists of carbs per major meal (i.e., breakfast, lunch and dinner) and 1 fist-sized portion for snacks and light meals.

Protein

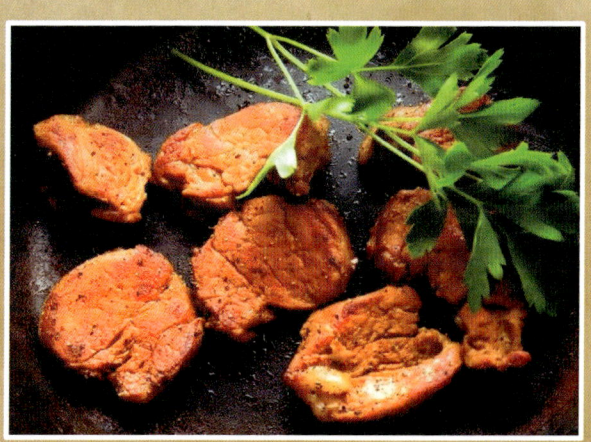

What it does - The basic building blocks of the body, utilised in the repair and rebuilding of tissue, organs and bone. Protein can also be used as energy in the absence of carbohydrates and fat.

Your approximate amount - Aim for a palm-sized portion of protein per major meal (i.e. breakfast, lunch and dinner). Half that amount for snacks and light meals.

Fats

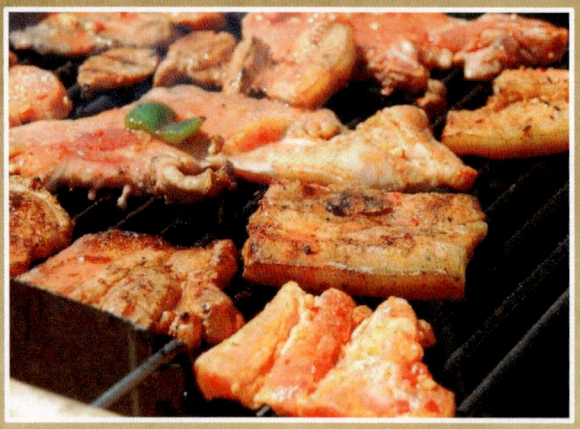

What they do - Fats primarily provide energy for the body, but they also have more uses in the body than any other food group, including protection and the uptake of many vitamins and minerals. Interestingly, fats are a major component in every cell in the body, bones and the brain.

Your approximate amount - Aim for a portion of fat roughly the size of the end of your thumb per major meal (i.e., breakfast, lunch and dinner) and half that for snacks and light meals.

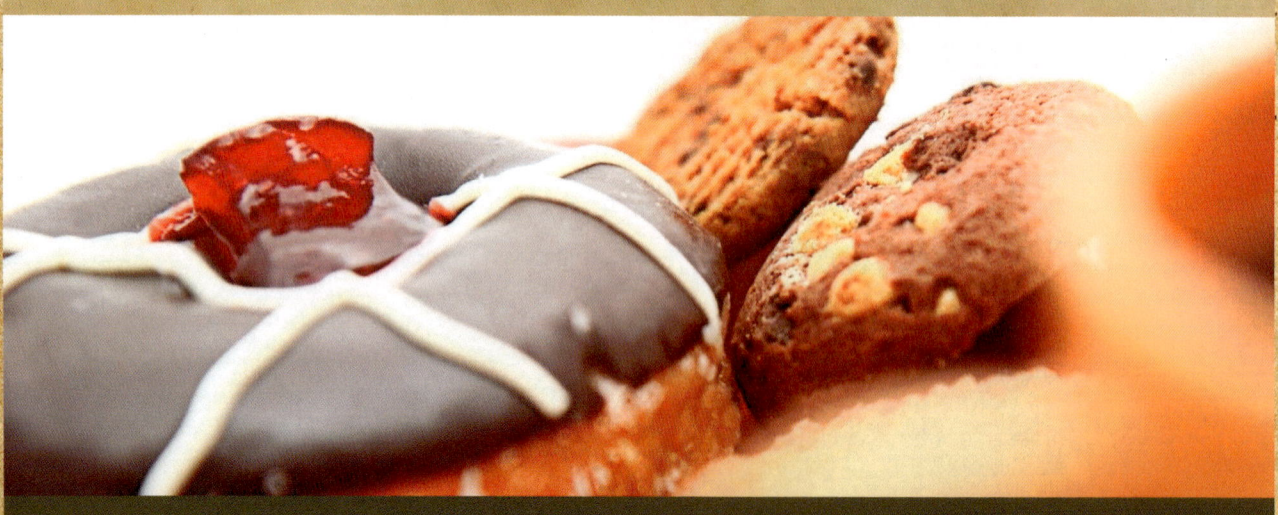

Remember that fats are your friend. Sugar is the enemy.

WATER

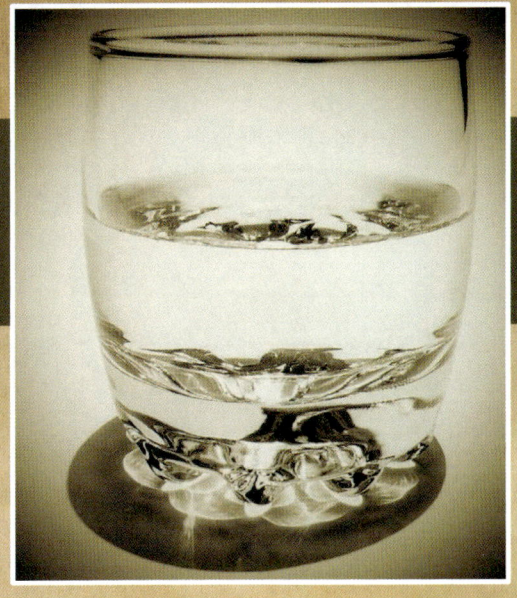

Though water is not considered to be a food group, it is a great ally in your quest for cleaner eating and the avoidance of overeating.

What it does - Water is involved in almost every function in the body, but you can also fool your body's satiety signals by partially filling the stomach with water prior to eating.

Your approximate amount - Consume no less than 3 litres of water per day to prevent dehydration, the slowing of your metabolism and to help dispel hunger. In hot climates or on warm days, increase your water intake to compensate. As an indication, your urine should be a pale straw colour.

Crash Prevention

We all know that feeling when we are so low on blood sugar that we are ready to kick the door off the fridge and bury our face in any sweet treat in there. Hitting the crash zone leads to one thing: the inability to make a smart food choice. Avoid hitting the crash zone with these three simple steps:

1. Eat regularly and aim for balanced meals every 2-3 hours to maintain blood sugar levels and prevent peaks and drops in blood sugar. Maintain breakfast, lunch and dinner as your larger main meals, but intersperse them with lighter meals of less quantity but exactly the same balance of nutrients.

2. Recognise the early symptoms of a crash. The ability to recognise the onset of a crash can hasten you to head for the shops before it is too late and you simply cannot fight off the craving for the sugary, fatty and salty food.

3. Predict when your blood sugar may start to waiver and prevent a crash by eating cleanly at the prescribed times to keep cravings at bay. Remember that when eating correctly, you should rarely feel hungry and will often need to prompt yourself to eat, as hunger and cravings are suppressed.

MAKE SMART CHOICES EASY

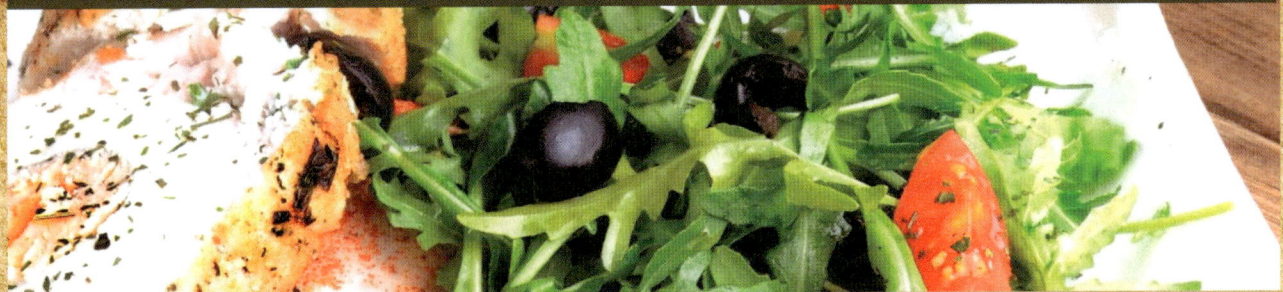

Today, poor choices are made incredibly easier. Crap food is usually cheaper, easier to get and is certainly more appealing due to the most relentless marketing known to man. Make smart choices easy to make by creating cheap, easy-to-create default meals that you can fall back on as well as identifying smart snack choices in all the regular shops and cafes you visit.

TACKLE SABOTAGE

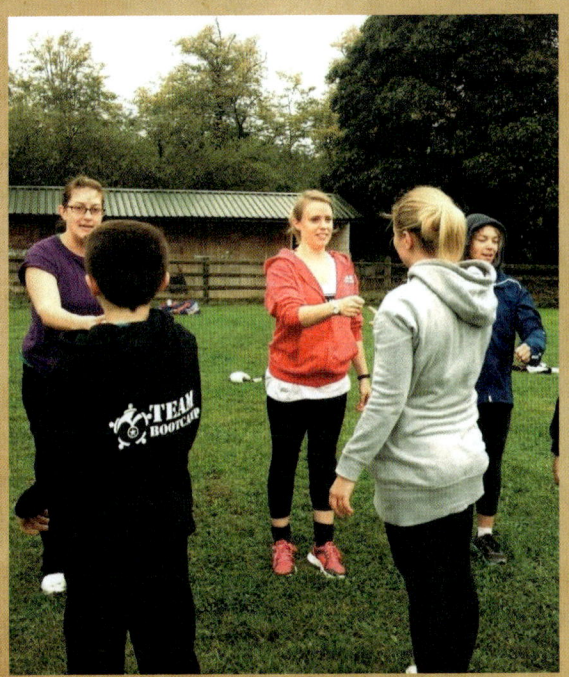

There are two types of people in your life: those that will help you with your weight loss and fitness goals, called aiders, and those that will do EVERYTHING in their power to stop you! I call the latter saboteurs, and they are the enemy in your quest for a fitter, healthier and leaner you! They will try everything from pulling on your heartstrings to laying their own food-related guilt on you. Take a minute to consider who the saboteurs are in your life.

In my experience, the easiest way to tackle saboteurs is to confront them. I suggest the following:

Mike, Tim, Sandra (or whatever their name is), as you know, I am trying to lose weight and get a little fitter, and I have identified you as a saboteur. I feel like you go out of your way to prevent me from truly being happy with myself. If you really want to help me don't sabotage my progress. Help me Instead.

Then, pause for as long as it takes and wait to hear what they have to say for themselves.

PREPARATION IS KEY

Prior preparation and planning prevents piss poor food choices. This takes little explanation, really. Planning and preparation really are keys to your success. Making a salad or grilling chicken for tomorrow takes time and effort, which, after a busy day at the office or running around after the kids, can be the last thing you want to do. But achieving your goals is going to take sacrifice and determination. You HAVE to plan ahead and prepare for the times you know that smart food is harder to get or inaccessible.

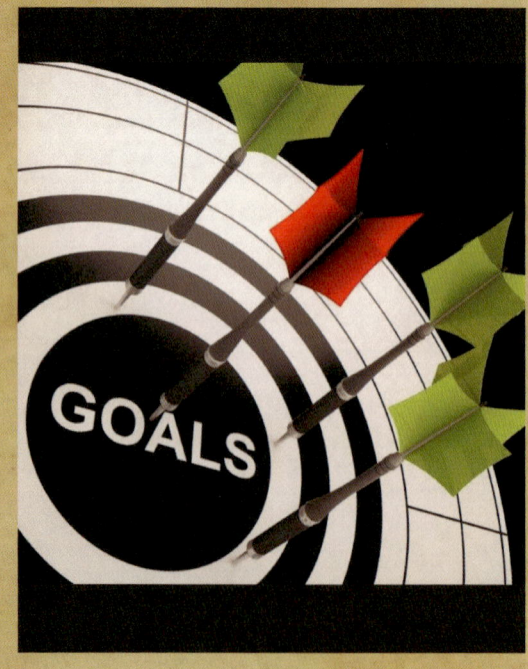

Make It a Habit

A very powerful thing to remember is the fact that it takes 21 days to form a new habit and a further 3 months to make that habit a lifelong change! Many people getting started on a fitness and fat loss programme fall off the wagon after 14 days or so because they take their eye off the ball. Just knowing that you need to push on for 21 days makes it much easier for you to succeed. It sets a target for you to meet, and once you reach it, things get that little bit easier.

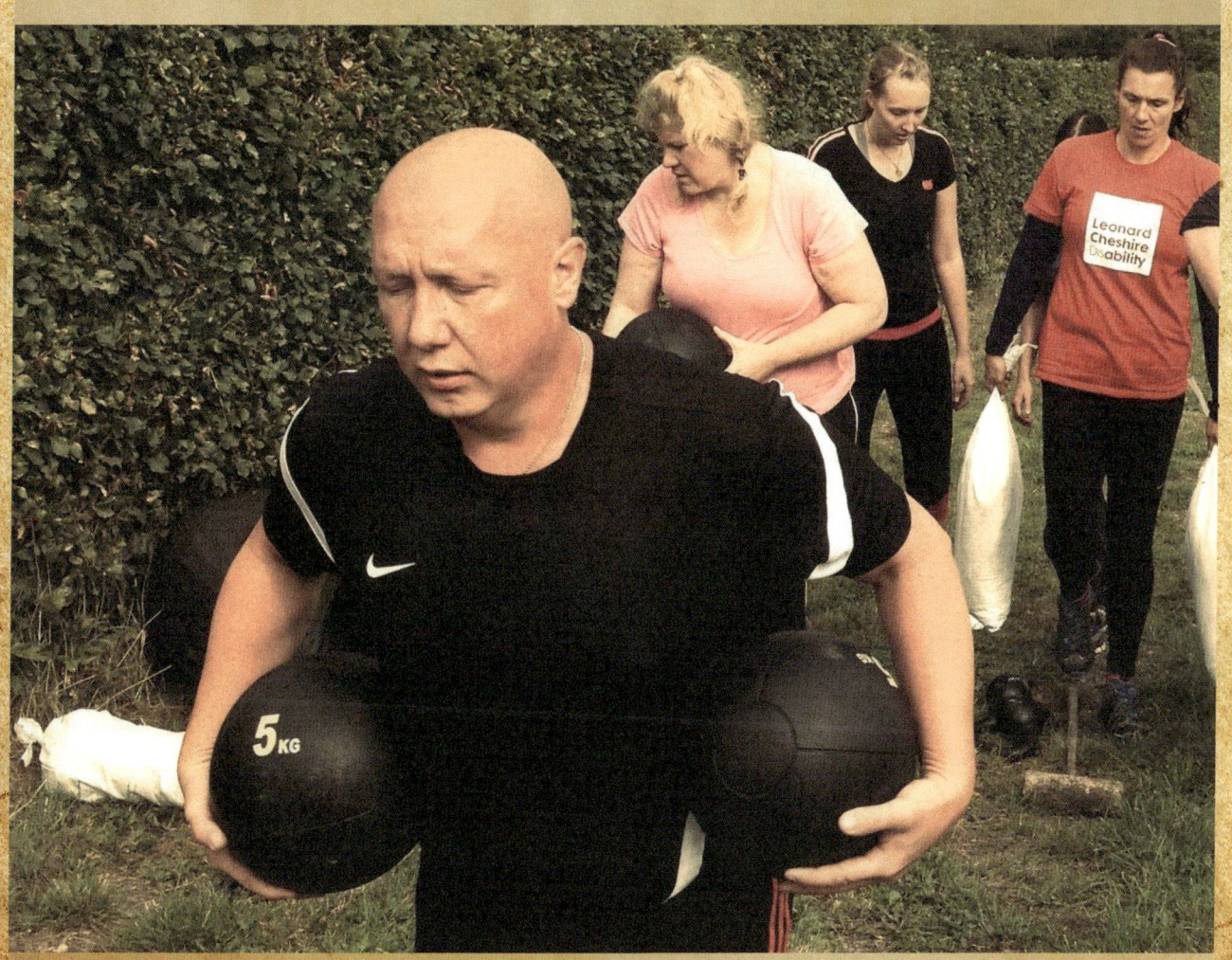

Section 2 - Introduction

At TEAM Boot Camp, we prescribe paleo nutrition because eating like our ancestors did prior to farming will mean you are fulfilling all of the tips and advice in the previous section without having to think about it. This section will give you a basic introduction to paleo nutrition and highlight the accepted foods. If you would like more information and resources to help you get started, visit paleotuckshop.com/resources.

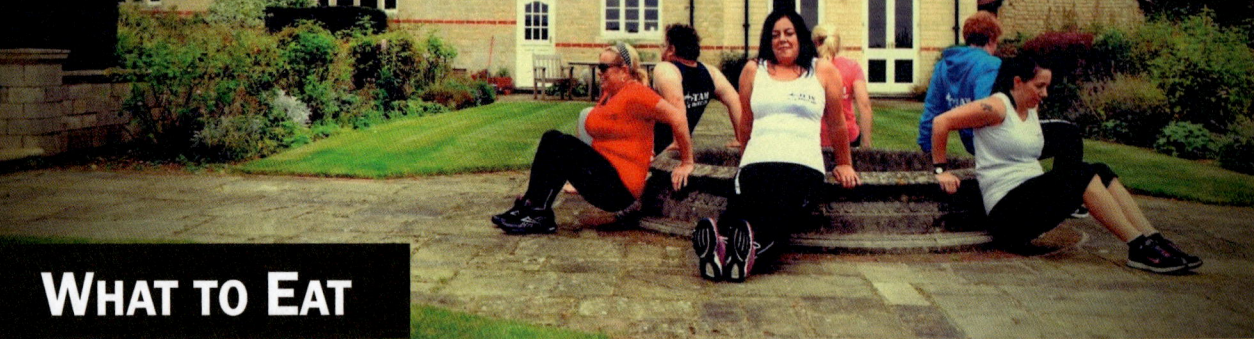

What to Eat

The mantra of good paleo nutrition is to eat lots of lean meats, fresh vegetables, some fruits, nuts and seeds. In basic terms, if you can catch it, kill it and grow it, you can eat it, but as with everything, there are some exceptions to that rule.

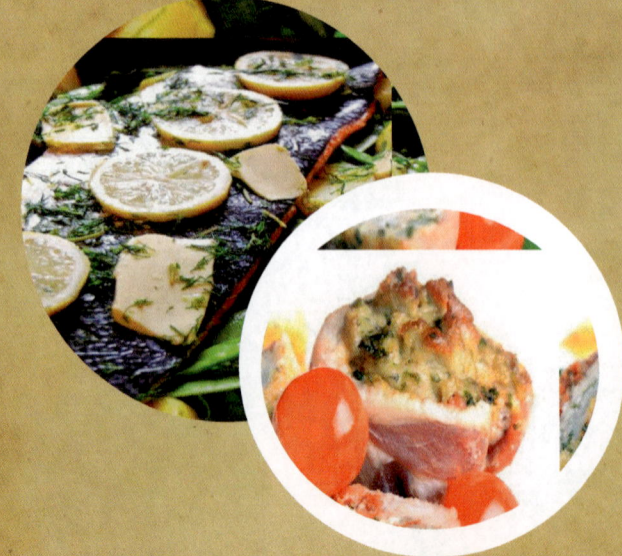

Here are some basic guidelines for your primal eating :

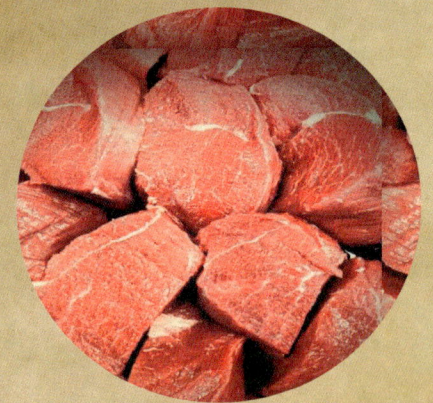

Meats – Eat as much as you want for breakfast, lunch and dinner with no extravagant cooking methods. Stick to broiling, baking, roasting, sautéing and browning lightly, all with no or little added fat. Drain off excess fat where possible.

When hungry or in doubt, lean meat is the most effective food group in reducing your appetite and boosting your metabolism to help burn stored fat.

Beef – Always trim any visible fat.

Steak	Top sirloin	Veal
Any other lean cut	Lean burgers	

Pork – Lean cuts only and always trim any visible fat.

Pork loin	Pork chops	Any other lean cut

Poultry – White meat, skin removed.

Chicken, ideally enriched omega 3 variety   Goose   Turkey breast

Offal

Beef, lamb, pork and chicken livers   Beef, lamb and pork tongues

Beef, lamb and pork marrow   Beef, lamb and pork sweetbreads

Other meats

Rabbit   Goat   Game

Fish

All unprocessed fish and shell fish, ideally wild caught

Eggs

Chicken, ideally enriched omega 3 variety   Goose   Duck

Fruits and Vegetables

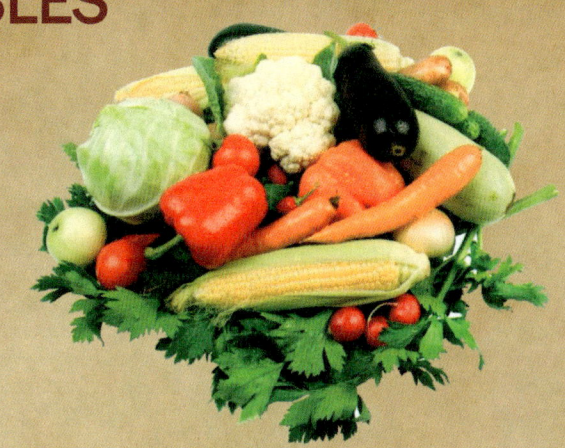

Ensure you max out on fresh, non-starchy vegetables during each meal along with moderate amounts of nuts, avocado, seeds and unsaturated oils (flaxseed, canola, olive oil and mustard seed).

Limit fruit to one or two portions a day, and definitely do not eat bananas unless you train like a dog and need to replace energy quickly following a heavy training session.

Remember, not all vegetables are good. Avoid high-carbohydrate, starchy tubers, such as potatoes and yams, and restrict the amount of sweet potatoes to 1 or 2 a week.

Nuts are very energy dense. If you are trying to lose weight, you should restrict your nut intake to around 4 ounces a day. Every nut (except walnuts) are very high in omega 6, and excessive intake should be counteracted with high-strength fish oil containing a high dosage of omega 3 to balance the omega 6 to omega 3 ratio.

Dried fruit should be eaten in very small amounts because of the high glycemic load, causing a rapid increase in the blood sugar level.

Fruits

Apple	Cranberries	Apricot	Figs
Avocado	Gooseberries	Blueberries	Grapefruit
Blackberries	Honeydew melon	Grapes	Guava
Cantaloupe	Kiwi	Lemon	Cassava melon
Lime	Nectarine	Pomegranate	Orange
Rasp-berries	Papaya	Rhubarb	Passion fruit
Star Fruit	Peaches	Strawberries	Pears
Tangerine	Persimmon	Watermelon	Pineapple
Plums			

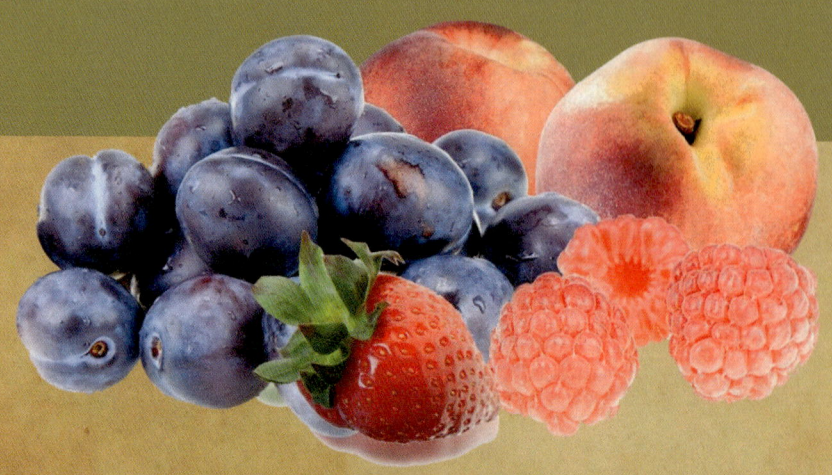

Vegetables

Artichoke	Mushrooms	Asparagus	Mustard greens
Beet greens	Onions	Beets	Parsley
Bell peppers	Parsnip	Broccoli	Peppers
Brussels sprouts	Pumpkin	Cabbage	Carrots
Radish	Cabbage	Cauliflower	Celery
Seaweed	Spinach	Cucumber	Squash (all kinds)
Tomato	Spring onions	Kale	Turnips
Suede	Watercress	Lettuce	

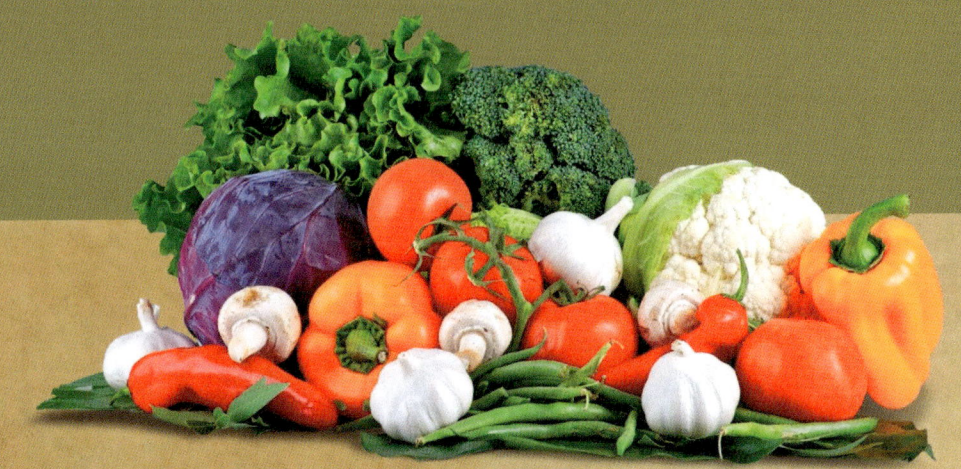

Nuts and seeds

Almonds	Pine nuts	Brazil nuts	Pistachios
Cashews	Pumpkin seeds	Chestnuts	Sesame seeds
Hazelnuts	Sunflower seeds	Macadamia nuts	Walnuts
Pecans			

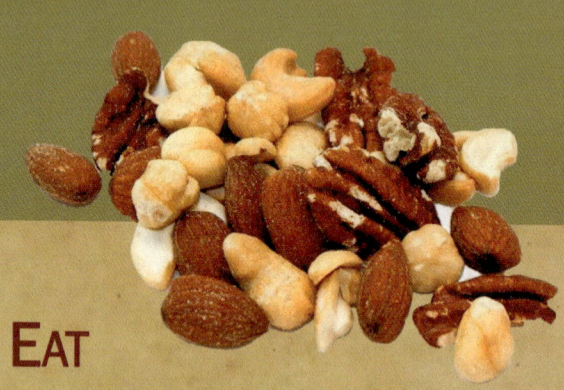

FOODS YOU CAN EAT IN MODERATION

Oils

- Olive oil
- Canola

Avocado
Coconut oil

Walnut

Flaxseed

Drinks

- Coffee   Tea   Fruit juice

Other food

- Dried fruit

FOODS TO AVOID

Avoid all processed foods and anything that starts with a capital letter, which suggests it's a brand name and not a real food.

Dairy products

- Butter   Cheese   Cream   Milk
- Dairy spreads   Powdered milk   Yoghurt   Ice cream

Cereal grains

Avoid the following foods or foods that contain the following:

- Barley   Corn   Millet   Oats
- Rice   Rye   Sorghum   Wheat

Grain-like seeds

- Quinoa   Buckwheat

Legumes

- All beans   Black-eyed peas   Chickpeas   Peanuts
- Lentils   Peas   Sugar snap peas   Peanut butter
- Miso   Soybeans and all soybean products, including tofu

Starchy vegetables

- Cassava root   Yams   Tapioca   Manioc
- Potatoes and all potato products

Foods high in salt

- Bacon   Processed meats   Pork rinds   Cheese
- Salami   Deli meats   Frankfurters   Ham
- Hot dogs   Ketchup   Pickled foods   Olives
- Salted nuts   Salted spices   Sausages   Smoked or dried fish and meat

- Virtually all canned meats and fish (unless you soak them)

Fatty meats

- Bacon
- Fatty cuts of pork

Fatty cuts of beef
Lamb chops

Chicken or turkey legs thigh, wings and skin
Cuts of lamb

Soft drinks

- All soft drinks   Energy drinks

Sweets

- All confectionary

    All refined sugars or foods high in refined sugar

- Cakes   Biscuits   Sweeteners   Most   honey

Breakfast

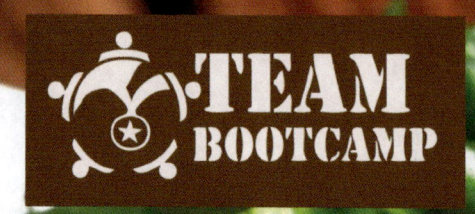

Granola

Serves – 4 - 6

Cooking time – 45 mins

Prep time - 20 mins

- Mix the chopped walnuts, macadamias, chopped almonds honey and cinnamon in a baking tray.
- Bake in an oven for 12 mins at 160°c. Remove and leave to cool.
- Place the flaked almonds and pumpkin seeds in another baking tray and bake in an oven for 10 mins at 160°c. Remove and leave to cool.
- Once all the ingredients have cooled, place into an airtight container, add the coconut and cranberries.
- Serve with unsweetened almond milk.

INGREDIENTS:

- 200g Flaked Almonds
- 200g Chopped walnuts
- 100g pumpkin seeds
- 200g Chopped macadamia nut
- 200g Chopped almonds
- 100g dried cranberries
- 100g sultanas
- 200g Desiccated coconut
- 100g Honey 2 tsp Cinnamon

TEAM BOOTCAMP

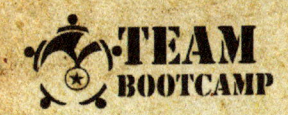

Tomato, bacon and rocket frittata

Serves - 4

Cooking time - 15 mins

Prep time - 10 mins

INGREDIENTS:

- Quarter the tomatoes and bake for 10 mins at 180°c
- Slice the bacon into thin strips
- Finely dice the onion
- Heat the olive oil in a frying pan before adding the onions. Add the bacon after a couple of minutes and cook for 5 mins before transferring to an oven dish.
- Beat the eggs and milk in a mixing bowl along with pinch of black pepper.
- Add the tomatoes, rocket to the oven dish before pouring the egg mix in and stirring.
- Place in a warm oven at 180°c for 15 mins.
- Slice into portions and serve with a small leafy salad.

- 1 small onion
- 4 plum tomatoes
- 4 slices of lean,
- Un-smoked bacon
- 40g rocket 6 free range eggs
- 150 ml of unsweetened almond milk
- 1 tsp olive oil Black pepper

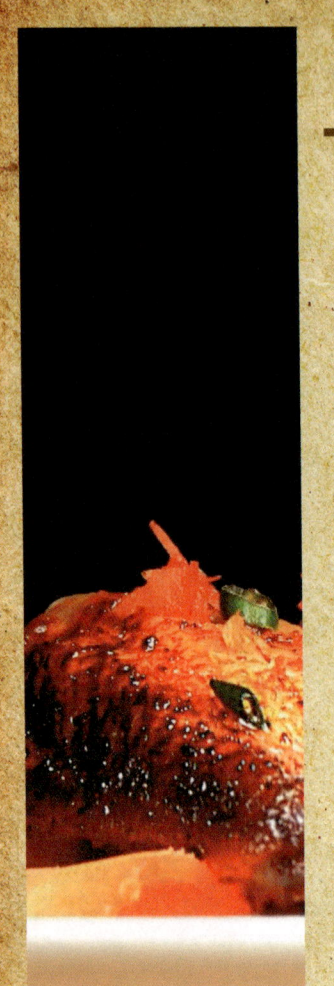

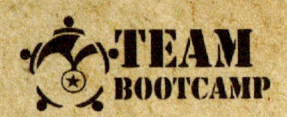

Avocado poached egg

Serves - 4

Cooking time – 15 mins

Prep time – 15 mins

INGREDIENTS:

- Halve the avocado and remove the stones.
- Place face down on a baking tray and bake for 15 mins at 200°c.
- To make the sauce – Add the yolks of two eggs, vinegar, lemon juice and bay leaf together in a glass bowl on a Bain Marie and whisk for 30-60 seconds.
- Pour in the oil whilst whisking until you have a good consistency, remove bay leaf and put sauce to one side.
- Poach the 4 eggs in a pan of hot (not boiling) water with a splash of vinegar for 4-5 mins.
- To serve place the egg on top of the avocado, flesh side up and drizzle with a little sauce.

- 1 Bay leaf
- 2 Avocados
- 6 Free range eggs
- 50ml extra virgin olive oil
- 1 lemon
- 1 tsp white wine vinegar
- Pinch of sea salt

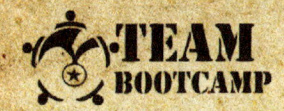

Bacon, spinach and red pepper omelette

Serves - 4

Cooking time – 6 mins

Prep time – 10 mins

INGREDIENTS:

- 1 onion
- 4 slices of lean unsmoked bacon
- 40g of spinach
- 1 red pepper
- 8 free range eggs
- Cracked black pepper
- Pinch of sea salt
- 1 tsp olive oil

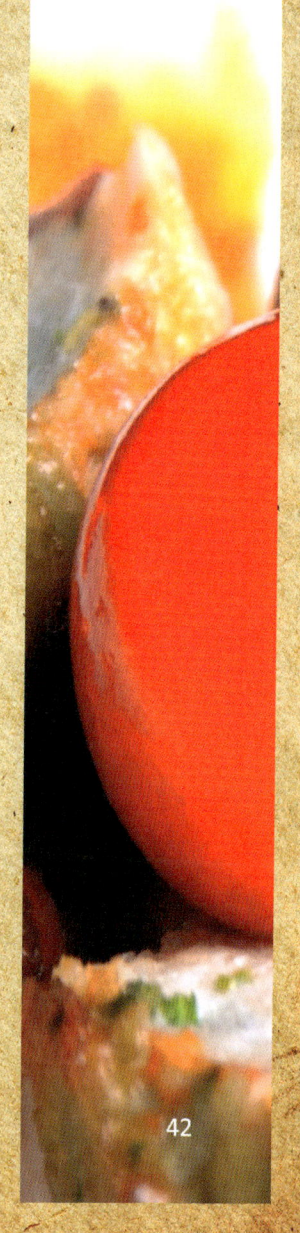

- Finely chop the onion, bacon and red pepper.
- Beat the eggs and the black pepper together in a bowl.
- Heat an omelette pan or small non-stick frying pan and sweat the onions.
- Add the bacon and red pepper and cook, stirring occasionally for 4-5 mins.
- Place the ingredients in a bowl and wipe the pan.
- Add a small drizzle of oil to the pan and heat. Add ¼ of the bacon and pepper mix. Cook for 30 secs and then add ¼ of the egg mix.
- Ensure the egg mix cooks evenly and after 30-40 secs, season with a pinch of salt and add 10g of spinach.
- Fold the omelette. The heat of the omelette will continue to cook the egg and spinach slightly.
- Plate and serve with a small leafy green salad.
- Repeat with a further 3 omelettes

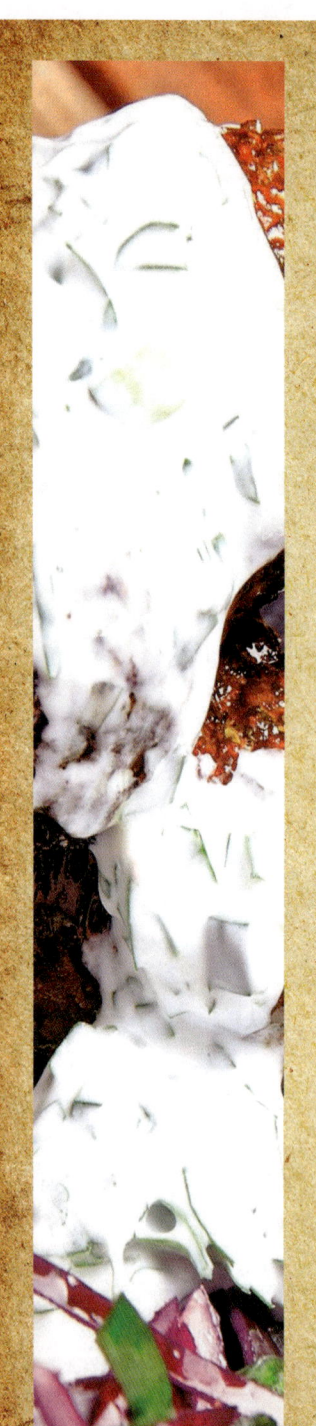

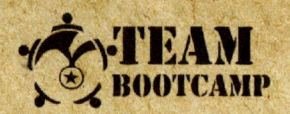

Date & honey pancakes

Serves - 4

Cooking time – 10 mins

Prep time – 10 mins

INGREDIENTS:

- Add almond milk, eggs and arrow root to a mixing bowl and whisk to an even consistency with no lumps or bumps.
- In a hot non-stick frying pan, add a small ladle of the batter mix. Sprinkle with chopped dates and cook for 1 minute.
- Flip and cook for a further 1 minute and serve.
- Repeat for additional pancakes

- 250g of arrow root – not Paleo, but worth it for pancakes
- 2 small free range eggs
- 150ml of unsweetened almond milk
- 60g of chopped dates
- 30g of Manuka honey
- Pinch of sea salt return 1 tsp olive oil

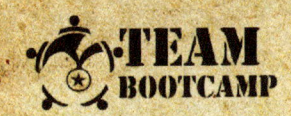

Smoked haddock Florentine on wilted baby spinach

Serves - 4

Cooking time - 20 mins

Prep time - 20 mins

INGREDIENTS:

- To make the sauce – Add the yolks of two eggs, vinegar, lemon juice and bay leaf together in a glass bowl on a Bain Marie and whisk for 30-60 seconds.
- Pour in the extra virgin olive oil while whisking and stir until you have an even consistency. Remove the bay leaf and place the bowl to one side.
- Place the haddock on an oven tray, season with a pinch of salt and pepper and bake at 180°c for 10 mins.
- In a hot pan, add the olive oil and spinach and stir for 2 -4 mins until wilted. Season with salt and pepper to taste and remove from the heat.
- Poach the eggs in hot (not boiling) water with a splash of white wine vinegar for 4-5 mins.
- To serve place the haddock onto the spinach with the eggs on top of the fish.
- Finish with a drizzle of sauce over the egg and a pinch of black pepper.

- 4 Smoked haddock fillets
- 1 bay leaf
- 80g of baby spinach
- 6 eggs
- 50ml of extra virgin olive oil
- 1 tsp of white wine vinegar
- 1 lemon
- Cracked black pepper
- Pinch of sea salt
- 1 tsp olive oil

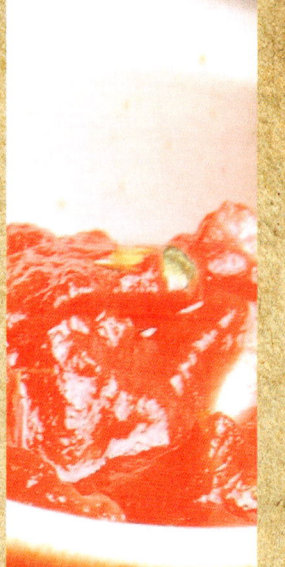

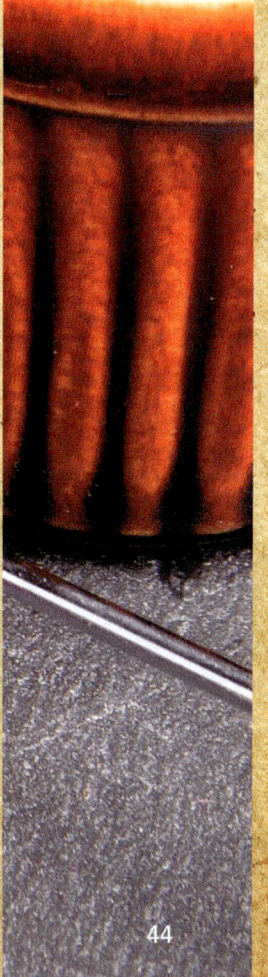

Snacks

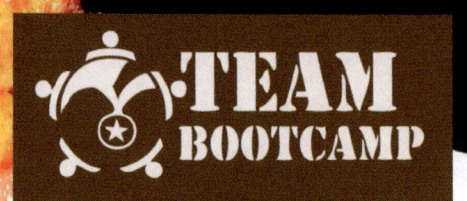

Cauliflower & Macadamia Humus

Serves - 6

Cooking time - 30 mins

Prep time - 30 mins

Resting - 1 hour

- Boil or steam the cauliflower until soft and leave to cool for a few minutes.
- Add the cauliflower and all the other ingredients to a food processor and blend until smooth.
- Allow to rest in the fridge for 1 hour before serving.

INGREDIENTS:

- 1 large cauliflower
- 100 g macadamia nuts
- 2 cloves of garlic
- 2 tbsp extra virgin olive oil
- 1 tsp cumin
- 1 lemon
- 1/2 tsp ground white pepper
- 1/4 tsp paprika

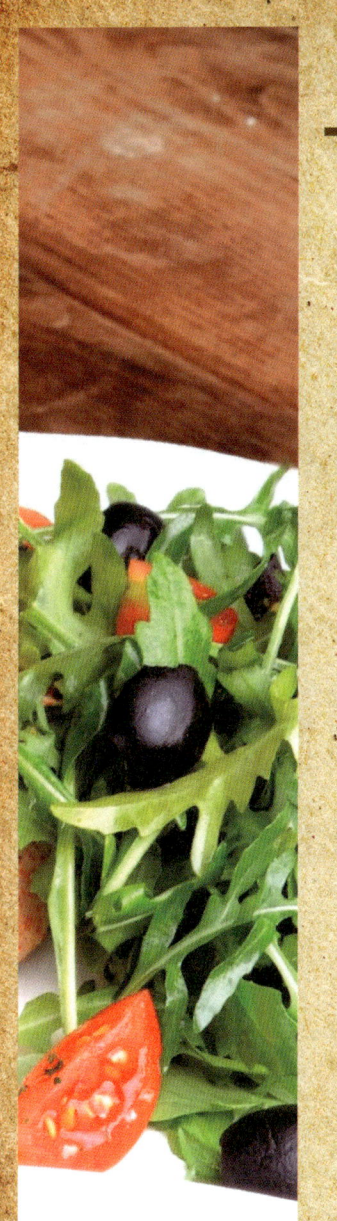

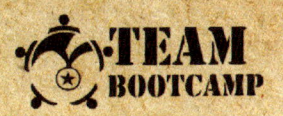

Sesame & Cranberry Flapjack

Serves - 6

Cooking time – 45 min

Prep time – 20 min

INGREDIENTS:

- Put honey, sesame seeds, walnuts, chopped and flaked almonds, sunflower seeds and cashew nuts in a pan and place on the stove on a low heat until honey has melted.
- Add cinnamon and cranberries and fold in.
- Put in a shallow tray lined with greaseproof paper.
- Bake at 150°C for 45 min.
- Press with a similar sized tray and allow to cool.

- 75 g set honey
- 50 g sesame seeds
- 100 g dried cranberries
- 125 g chopped walnuts
- 125 g flaked almonds
- 75 g sunflower seeds
- 100 g chopped cashew nut
- 100 g chopped almonds
- 1 tsp cinnamon

TEAM BOOTCAMP

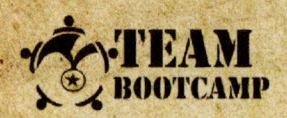

Chicken Nuggets

Serves - 4

Cooking time - 25 mins

Prep time - 20 mins

INGREDIENTS:

- Cut chicken breasts into bite sized chunks.
- Put the arrowroot, 2 eggs (beaten) and ground almonds into 3 different dishes for coating.
- Zest 1/4 lemon and add to almonds.
- Add chopped sage and pinch cracked to almonds.
- Coat chicken by putting it into the arrowroot and egg mix and the coat in the almond mix. Place on a tray and leave in a fridge for 30 minutes.
- With a hot pan add the oil and fry the nuggets turning them until they are a golden brown colour.
- Put in the oven at 180°C for 12 minutes.

- 1 teaspoon olive oil
- 2 chicken breasts
- 3 tablespoons arrowroot
- 200 g ground almonds
- 2 eggs
- Cracked black pepper
- 1 lemon
- Sage

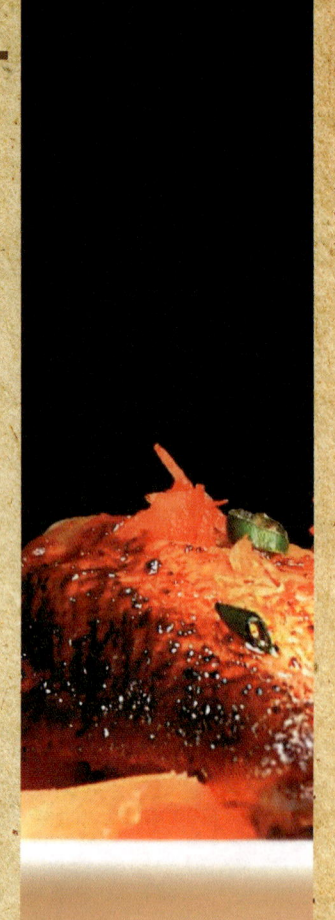

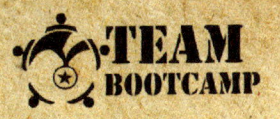

Chocolate Chip Cookies

Serves - 6

Cooking time – 20 mins

Prep time – 15 mins

INGREDIENTS:

- Mix all ingredients together thoroughly.
- Roll the mix into 6 equally sized balls and press flat, about 7-8 mm thick
- Line a tray with greaseproof paper
- Bake at 170°C for 20 minutes
- Allow to cool slightly so they firm up

- 125 g arrowroot
- 250 g ground almonds
- 50 g honey
- 2 eggs
- 50 g 80% or over dark chocolate (chopped)

Trail Mix

Serves - 4

Prep time – 10 min

INGREDIENTS:

- Mix all ingredients together, don't cook or bake.
- Store in a sealed container in a dry place.
- Serve approx. 55-65g per serving.

- 75g whole almonds
- 30g chopped walnuts
- 30g chocolate cashew nuts
- 30g pumpkin seed
- 30g sunflower seeds
- 30g sultanas
- 30g chopped dates

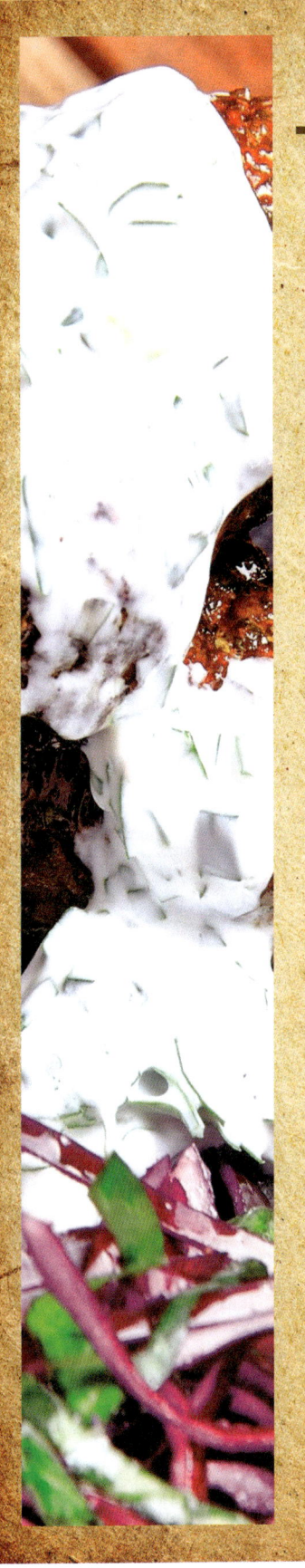

TEAM BOOTCAMP

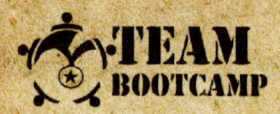

Dark Chocolate & Pistachio Brownie

Serves - Approx. 20 brownies
Cooking time – 20 mins
Prep time – 10 mins

INGREDIENTS:

- Place a heatproof dish on top of a pan of boiling water. Break the chocolate up and melt it using the steam.
- Add the rest of the ingredients and mix thoroughly.
- Place in a pre-heated oven at 200°C for approx 20 mins.

- 1 tbs Coca powder
- 200g 75-90% chocolate
- 125ml honey
- 6 eggs
- 200g ground almonds
- 1 tbs orange zest (optional)
- 50g raisins (optional)

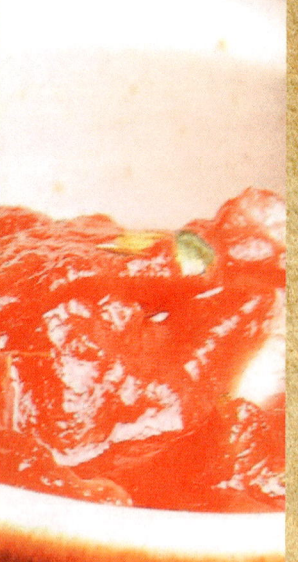

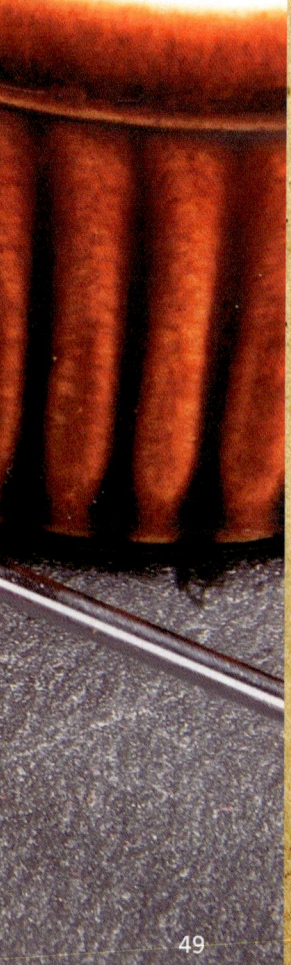

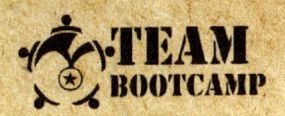

Carrot Cake

Serves - 4

Cooking time – 35 mins

Prep time – 20 mins

INGREDIENTS:

- Grate carrots.
- Put arrowroot, honey, baking powder, almonds, cinnamon in a bowl and mix.
- Beat eggs in a separate bowl and add to mix.
- Add grated carrot and olive oil and mix together.
- Line a cake tin with greaseproof paper.
- Bake at 160°C for 25 minutes then at 140°C for 10 more minutes.

- 275 g carrots
- 100 g arrowroot
- 50 g honey
- 1 teaspoon baking powder
- 50 g ground almonds
- 2 teaspoons cinnamon
- 3 eggs
- 1 tablespoon olive oil

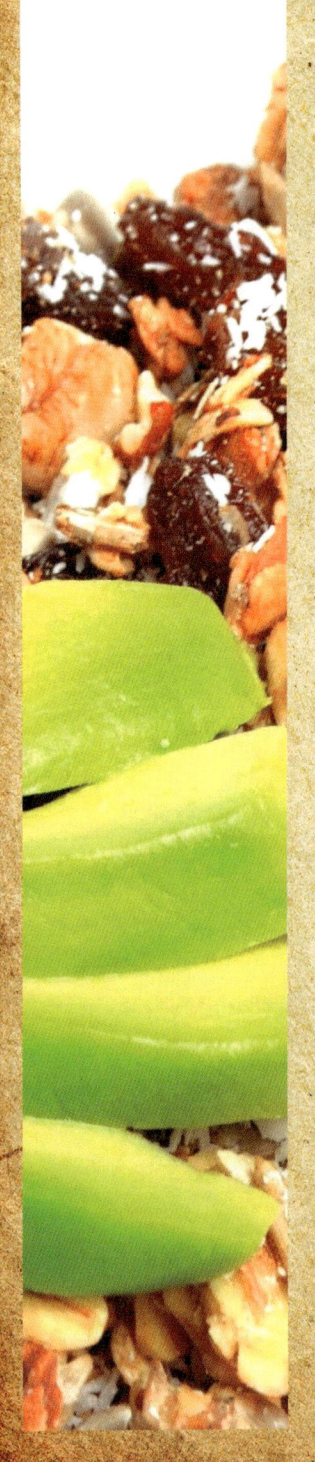

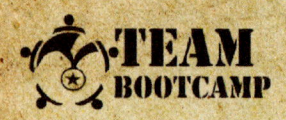

Coconut & Pineapple Pot

Serves - 4

Resting – 7-8 hours

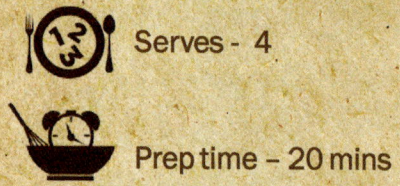

Prep time – 20 mins

INGREDIENTS:

- Put milk, coconut cream and honey in a pan on a low heat to warm through on the stove.
- Remove from heat before it starts to boil.
- While the hot mix cools for 10 minutes soak gelatin in cold water until soft.
- Remove gelatin from water and squeeze out any excess water.
- Stir the gelatin into milk mixture until dissolved.
- Pour the mix into ramekins or small cups and place in fridge for 7-8 hours to set.
- Garnish with pineapple pieces when fully cooled.

- 600 ml unsweetened almond milk
- 160 ml tin of coconut cream
- 70 g honey
- 5 gelatin leaves
- 100 g pineapple pieces

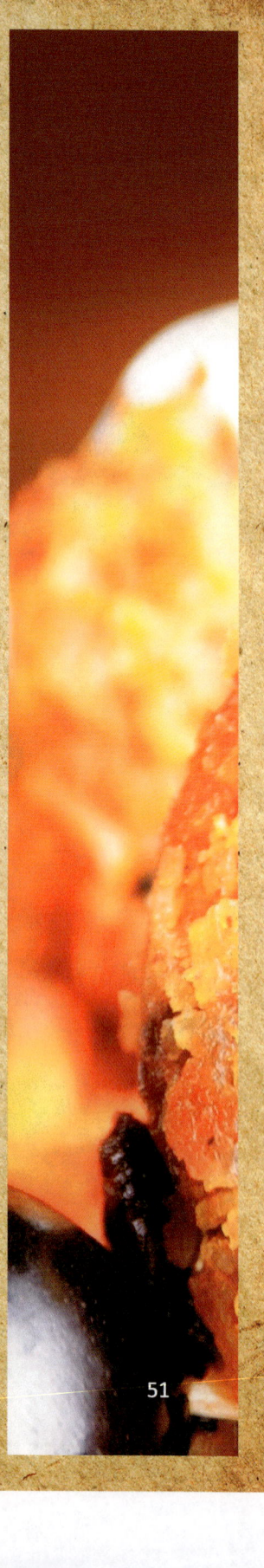

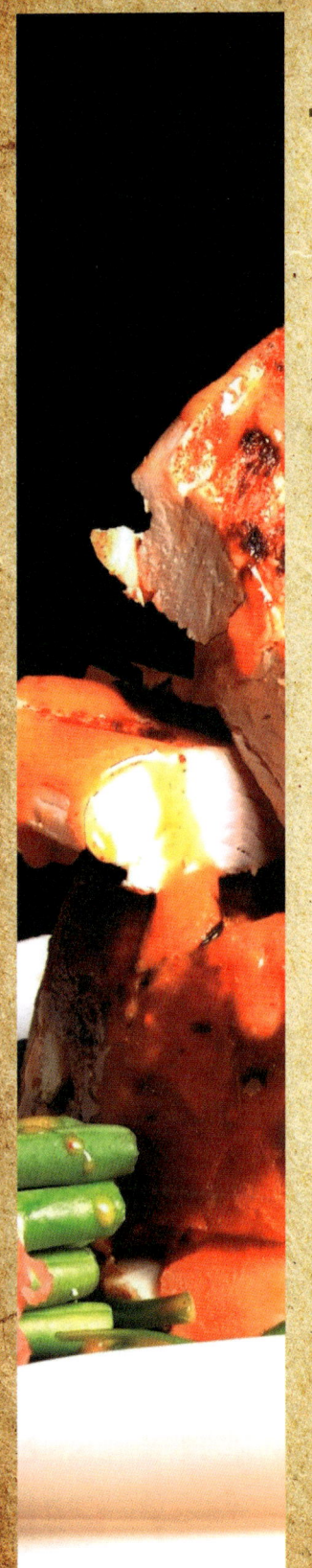

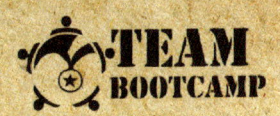

Chive & Cayenne Stuffed Egg

Serves – 1 egg = 1

Cooking time – 10 mins

Prep time – 15 mins

INGREDIENTS:

- Hard boil the eggs.
- Place under running cold water until fully cooled.
- Peel eggs and remove yolk and place in small bowl.
- Add chopped chives, cayenne pepper, olive oil and black pepper to yolks and mix until smooth.
- With a piping bag or teaspoon works the yolk mix back into the cooked egg white.
- Serve with rocket or salad (no dressing).

- 20-30 g rocket
- 4 eggs
- Fresh chives or 1 teaspoon dried chives
- 1/4 teaspoon cayenne pepper
- 1/2 teaspoon extra virgin olive oil
- Cracked black pepper (pinch)

TEAM BOOTCAMP

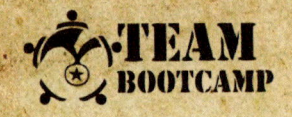

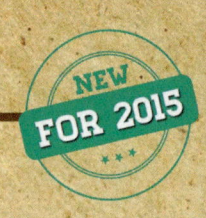

NEW FOR 2015

Spiced Coconut Bites

Serves - 6

Cooking time – 20 mins

Prep time – 20 mins

INGREDIENTS:

- Cook the chicken at 180°c in the oven for 20 mins then chill completely.
- Finely chop the chilli and garlic and slice the chicken breast into thin slices.
- Mix the coconut yoghurt, all the spices, garlic, chilli and a pich of chopped coriander in a mixing bowl.
- Add the chicken to the bowl and stir in.
- Separate 6 leaves from the gem lettuce and wash.
- Once dry, spoon on the chicken evenly between the leaves.
- Finish with a pinch of black pepper and sprinkle of chopped coriander then serve.

- 1 chicken breast
- 100g coconut milk yoghurt
- 1 tsp paprika
- ½ tsp cumin
- ½ tsp turmeric
- 1 clove of garlic
- 1 small green chilli
- Small bunch of coriander
- Pinch of cracked black pepper
- 1 baby gem lettuce

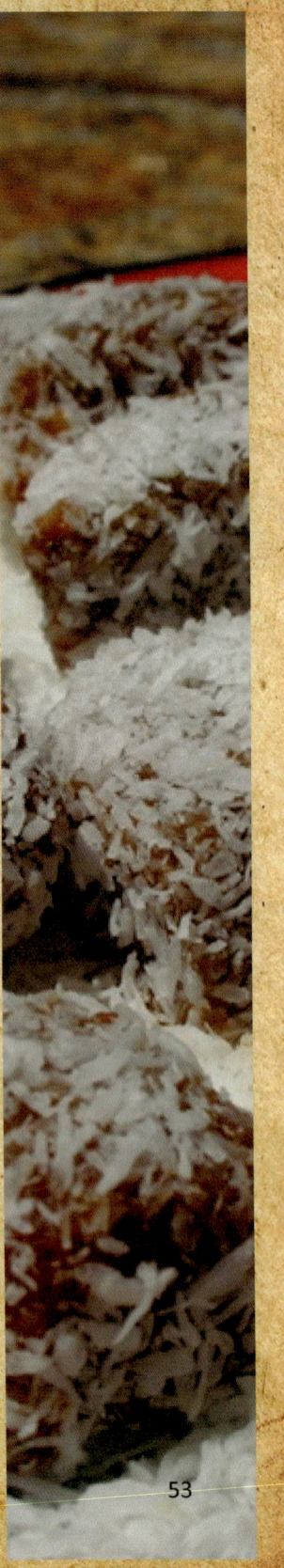

NEW FOR 2015

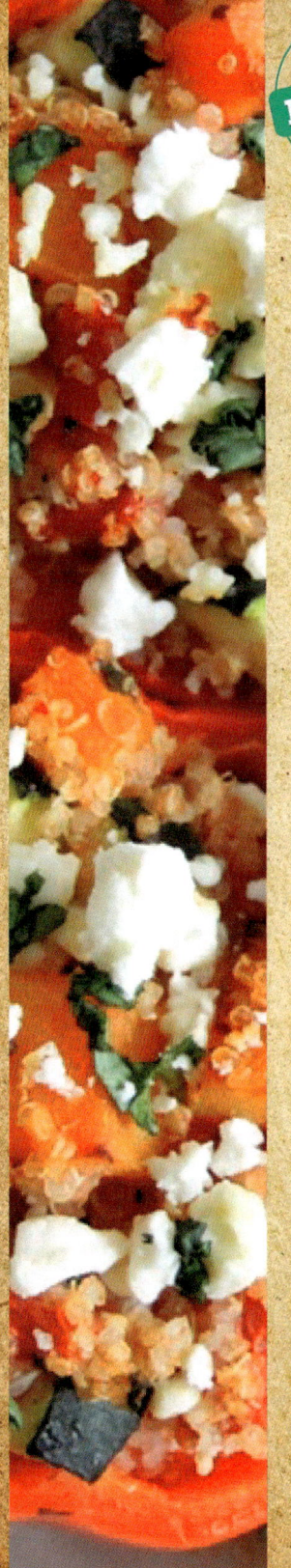

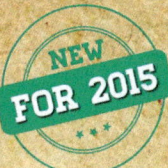

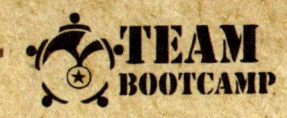

TEAM BOOTCAMP

Feta and Basil Stuffed Tomatoes

Serves - 4

Cooking time – 20 mins

Prep time – 10 mins

INGREDIENTS:

- Cut the beef tomatoes in half and spoon out the seeds.
- Finely chop the shallot and garlic.
- Quarter the cherry tomatoes and shred the basil.
- Heat the olive oil and sweat the shallot and garlic for 3-5 mins.
- Add the cherry tomatoes. Cook for 3 mins and then remove from the heat.
- Stir in half the basil and spoon the mixture into each half of the tomato.
- Crumble the feta on top and bake in the oven for 12 mins at 180°c.
- Remove from the oven and allow to cool. Finish by sprinkling the remainder of the basil on top, season with black pepper and serve.

- 2 Beef tomatoes
- 20g Feta cheese
- 1 small shallot
- 1 clove of garlic
- 6 cherry tomatoes
- 1 tsp tomato puree
- 1 tsp olive oil
- Small bunch of basil
- Pinch of cracked black pepper

TEAM BOOTCAMP

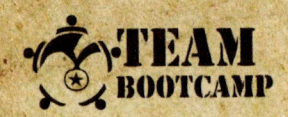

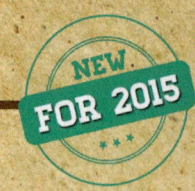

NEW FOR 2015

Bacon, Tomato and Egg Muffins

Serves - 6

Cooking time – 20 mins

Prep time – 10 mins

INGREDIENTS:

- 6 cherry tomatoes
- 4 eggs
- 2 slices of bacon
- 2 spring onions
- 1 bunch of chives
- Pinch of cracked black pepper
- 1 tsp olive oil

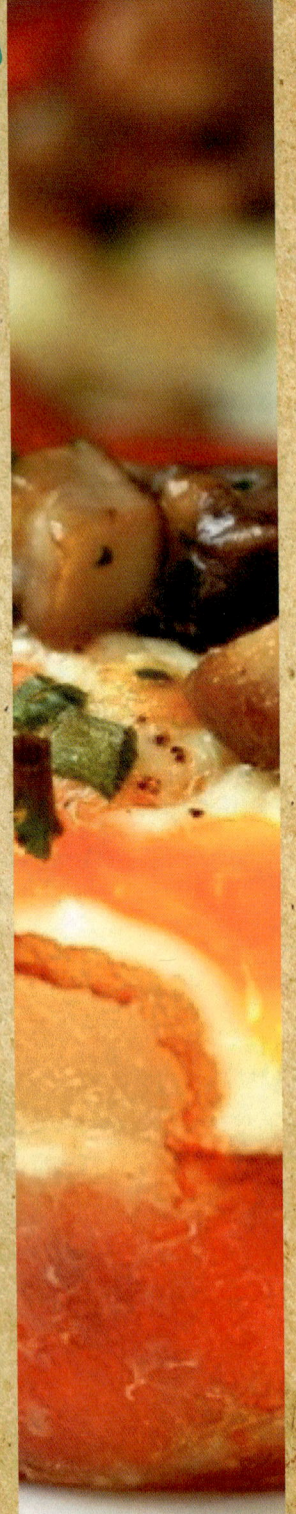

- Slice the bacon, spring onion and chives.
- Quarter the cherry tomatoes.
- Crack the egg into a bowl and beat with a pinch of black pepper.
- Heat a little oil in a pan and cook the bacon until crispy then add the spring onion and cook for 2 mins.
- Put the tomatoes and chives into the pan, stir then remove from the heat.
- Spoon the mixture evenly between 6 muffin cases.
- Pour the egg mix evenly over each of the mixes.
- Cook in an oven at 200°c for 15 mins and remove.
- Allow to rest for 5 minutes before serving.

Lamb

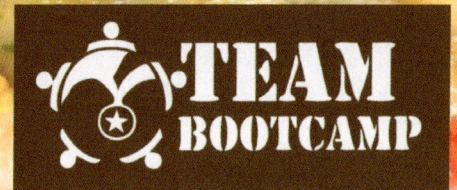

Rosemary & Garlic Lamb with Aubergine and Courgette Stack

Serves - 4

Cooking time - 120 mins

Prep time - 40 mins

INGREDIENTS:

- Brown the lamb shanks in a very hot large pan and move to a deep oven dish.
- Roughly chop the garlic, onion, carrots and half the lemon.
- Place into the oven dish with the lamb and add the stock and put in the oven at 180°C for 120 min.
- Peel and dice the butternut squash into 1 cm pieces.
- Slice and wash the leeks.
- Quarter the figs and cover with the honey on an oven tray.
- On a large oven tray add the butternut squash and leek season with a pinch of salt and pepper and a splash of olive oil.
- Put in the oven for 45 min at 180°C.
- Put the figs in the oven for 20 min at 180°C.
- Once all is cooled serve with the vegetables on the bottom then lamb and finish with the figs and honey.

- 4 lamb shanks
- 2 lts lamb or vegetable stock
- Bunch rosemary
- 1 bulb garlic
- 1 onion
- 2 carrots
- 1 lemon
- Olive oil
- 2 butternut squash
- 3-4 leeks
- 4 figs
- 35 g honey
- Cracked black pepper
- Pinch sea salt

TEAM BOOTCAMP

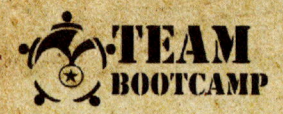

Braised Lamb Shank on Roasted Butternut Squash & Leek with Honey Roasted Figs

Serves - 4

Cooking time - 120 mins

Prep time - 40 mins

INGREDIENTS:

- Brown the lamb shanks in a very hot large pan and move to a deep oven dish.
- Roughly chop the garlic, onion, carrots and half the lemon.
- Place into the oven dish with the lamb and add the stock and put in the oven at 180ºC for 120 min.
- Peel and dice the butternut squash into 1 cm pieces.
- Slice and wash the leeks.
- Quarter the figs and cover with the honey on an oven tray.
- On a large oven tray add the butternut squash and leek season with a pinch of salt and pepper and a splash of olive oil.
- Put in the oven for 45 min at 180ºC.
- Put the figs in the oven for 20 min at 180ºC.
- Once all is cooled serve with the vegetables on the bottom then lamb and finish with the figs and honey.

- 4 lamb shanks
- 2 lts lamb or vegetable stock
- Bunch rosemary
- 1 bulb garlic
- 1 onion
- 2 carrots
- 1 lemon
- Olive oil
- 2 butternut squash
- 3-4 leeks
- 4 figs
- 35 g honey
- Cracked black pepper
- Pinch sea salt

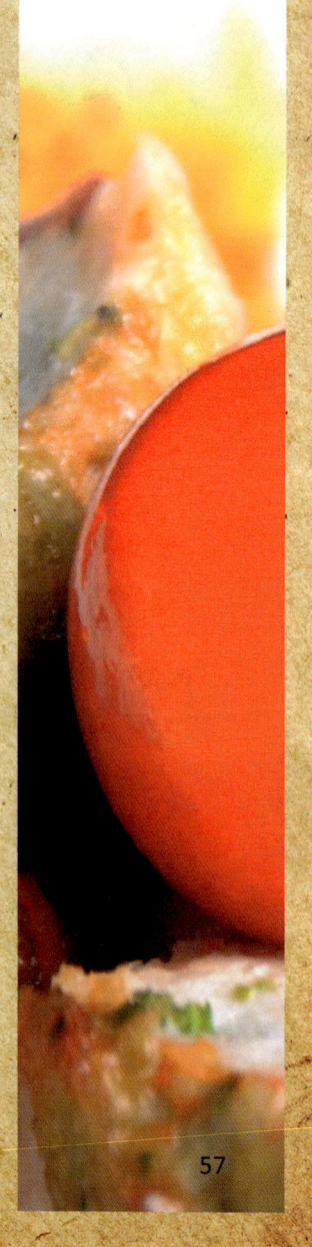

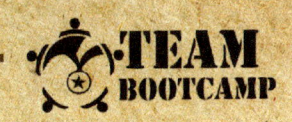

Paleo Lamb Tagine

Serves - 4

Cooking time - 90 mins

Prep time - 30 mins

INGREDIENTS:

- Using a hot pan brown the lamb and put in an oven-proof dish.
- Finely chop the onion, garlic and chilli and sweat in the same pan and add to lamb.
- To the lamb add the apricot, stock, cumin, star anise, cloves, cinnamon, turmeric and tomato puree, cover and put in the oven at 190ºC for 25 min.
- Peel and chop the butternut squash and slice the red and green pepper and add to the tagine, return to the oven for 60 min.
- Once cooked finish with some toasted chopped macadamia nuts and chopped coriander.

- 12 dried apricots
- 600 g diced lamb
- 1 onion
- 2 cloves garlic
- 750 mL lamb stock
- 2 medium chilli
- 1 tsp. cumin
- 1 star anise
- 1/2 tsp. cinnamon
- 2 cloves
- 1 red pepper
- 1 green pepper
- 1 tbsp. tomato puree
- Bunch coriander
- 1 butternut squash
- 50 g macadamia nuts
- 1 tsp. turmeric

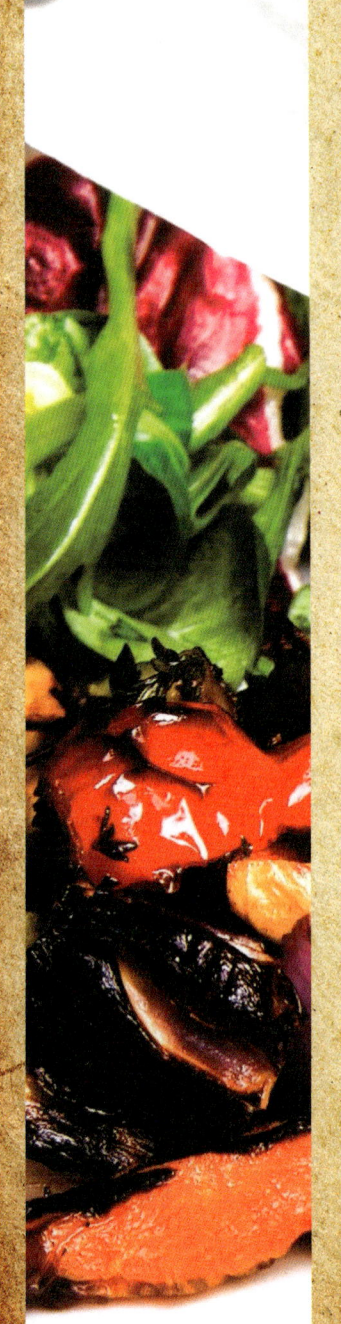

TEAM BOOTCAMP

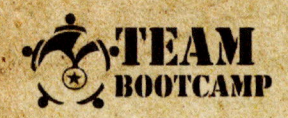

Rack of Lamb, Sweet Potato Rosti, with Red Current & Thyme Sauce

Serves - 4

Cooking time - 30 mins

Prep time - 30 mins

INGREDIENTS:

- Peel and grate the sweet potato, add to a bowl with the arrowroot, pinch of salt and black pepper.
- Form into 4 rosti's and squeeze out any liquid and let rest in fridge.
- Roughly chop the red and green peppers and put in a tray with the artichoke, few sprigs of thyme, 3 crushed garlic cloves, oil and pinch black pepper and roast at 180ºC for 35 min
- Pan fry the rostis and oven at 180ºC for 30 min.
- Using a very hot pan seal the rack of lamb and put on a try and season and cook at 180ºC for 15 min and allow to rest for 6-9 min.
- In the same pan deglaze with the stock, add zpuree, red currents and few sprigs of thyme.
- Reduce the sauce to desired thickness and season with a pinch of salt and pepper.
- To serve place the vegetables on a plate, slice the lamb between the bones and fan over, drizzle the sauce around and serve.

- 4 small trimmed racks of lamb
- 2 large sweet potatoes
- 2 red peppers
- 2 green peppers
- 1 can of artichoke hearts
- 100 g red currents
- Bunch thyme
- 3 cloves garlic
- 1 tbsp. arrowroot
- 1 tbsp. olive oil
- 500 mL lamb stock
- 1 tsp. tomato puree
- Cracked black pepper
- Sea salt

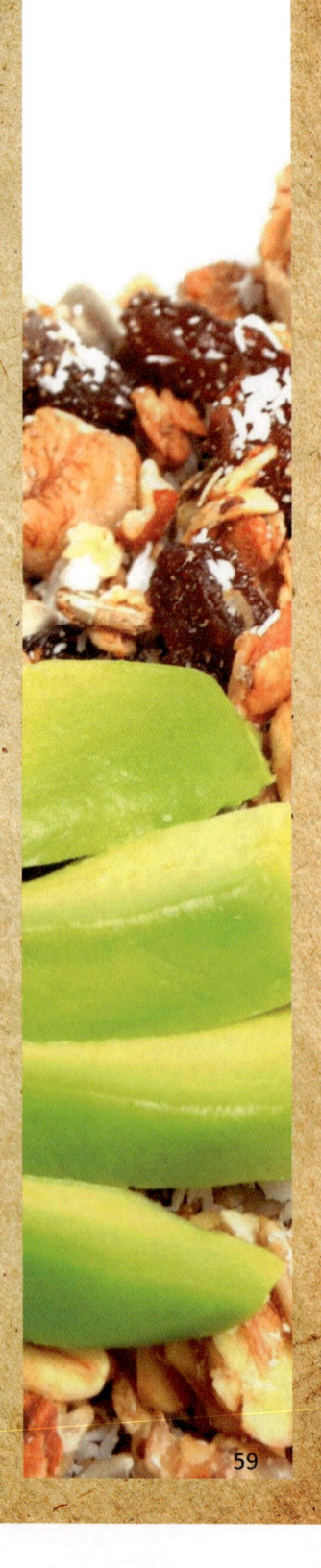

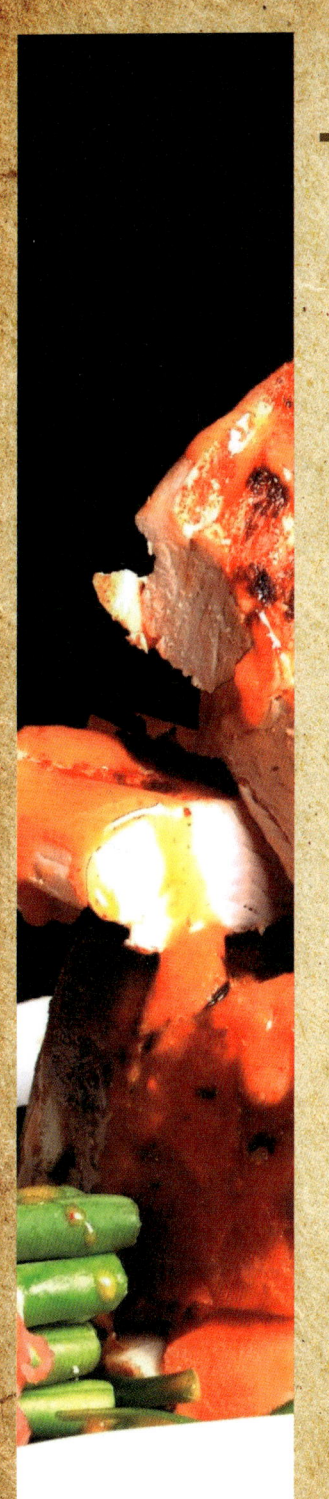

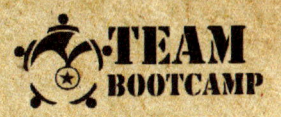

Lamb Kofta with Tzatziki with Spiced Tomato, Shallots & Minted Cabbage

Serves - 4

Cooking time - 30 mins

Prep time - 45 mins

INGREDIENTS:

- Finely chop the onion, 1/2 chillis and small handful of coriander and add to lamb mince.
- In a hot pan add cumin seeds, mustard seeds and cook dry for 4-5 min, cool and add to mince.
- Add to the mince lemon zest, few springs thyme, ground cumin, paprika, turmeric, pinch salt and pepper.
- Mix the mince and form into 8 sausage shape kebabs and put on a skewer, seal on a hot pan and oven for 30 min at 180°C.
- Peel and quarter the shallots, pan fry with some chili finely chopped and roast at 180°C for 20 min.
- Slice the cabbage finely and add to a mixing bowl with 6-8 chopped mint leaves, 1 tsp olive oil, pinch of salt and pepper and juice of 1/2 lemon, mix and put in the fridge.
- For the tzatziki, de-seed and finely dice the cucumber, chop 6-8 mint leaves and add to yoghurt with the juice of 1/2 lemon and pinch salt and pepper.
- To serve, put the shallot and tomatoes on the plate and kebabs on top with the tzatziki spooned on the side.

- 2 tsp olive oil
- 600 g lamb mince
- 2 medium onions
- 1/4 cucumber
- 100 g goats yoghurt
- 1 lemon
- 4 small bunches vine on cherry tomatoes
- 4 large shallots
- 1/2 white or red cabbage
- Bunch mint
- Bunch lemon thyme
- Bunch coriander
- 1 teaspoon cumin seeds
- 1 teaspoon mustard seeds
- 2 medium chilis
- 1/2 teaspoon ground cumin
- 1 teaspoon paprika
- 1 teaspoon turmeric
- 1 teaspoon ground black
- Pepper
- Pinch salt

Beef

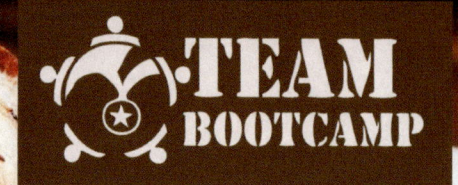

Braised Steak with Parsnip & Baby Onions

Serves - 4

Cooking time - 120 mins

Prep time - 40 mins

INGREDIENTS:

- 4 x 6 oz rump or braising steaks
- 2 large parsnips
- 250 g baby onion or baby leeks
- 500 mL beef stock
- Bunch rosemary
- 3 garlic cloves
- 1 tsp olive oil
- 1 tbsp tomato puree
- Cracked black pepper
- Pinch sea salt

- Peel and roughly chop the parsnip.
- Finely chop the garlic.
- Using a hot non-stick pan seal of the steaks for 4-5 minutes on both sides in the olive oil.
- Remove the steaks and put in an oven-proof dish.
- Using the same pan put in the parsnips and baby onions and colour for 2 minutes and add to the oven dish with the steaks.
- Add a few sprigs of rosemary and pour over the stock.
- Add a pinch of black pepper and the tomato puree gently stir in.
- Place in the oven at 180 º C for 100 min.
- Remove the rosemary stalks and then season with sea salt to taste.

Serve on its own or with sweet potato mash or seared savoy cabbage.

TEAM BOOTCAMP

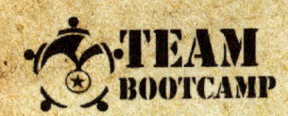

Meatballs & Ribbon Vegetables

Serves - 4
Cooking time - 45 mins
Prep time - 60 mins

INGREDIENTS:

- For the meatballs - Finely chop the onions and sweat in a pan until soft and allow to cool.
- Finely chop the garlic and sage.
- In a bowl mix the mince, onions, sage, garlic, tomato puree and nutmeg together and roll into bite sized balls.
- For the sauce roughly chop the onion, celery and garlic and using a large pan sweat of for 10 min.
- Add the chopped tomatoes, tomato puree and pinch of black pepper and simmer for 20 minutes.
- To finish the sauce add the honey, stir and then blend until smooth.
- Chop the basil finely and add to sauce with salt to taste.
- For the vegetables - Peel the butternut squash and using a vegetable peeler slice the butternut squash, carrots and courgettes.
- Cook the meatballs in the oven at 200°C for 20 min and add to the sauce.
- Heat a pan of water until boiling before adding the vegetables. Cook the vegetables for no longer than 90 secs.

Meatballs

- 600 g lean steak mince
- 2 onions
- Sage
- 2 garlic cloves
- 1 tbsp. tomato puree
- 1/2 tsp. ground nutmeg

Sauce

- 10 tomatoes or 2 tins chopped tomatoes
- 150 g tomato puree
- 1 onion
- 1 celery stick
- 2 cloves garlic
- 1 tsp. honey
- Bunch basil
- Pinch sea salt
- Pinch cracked black pepper

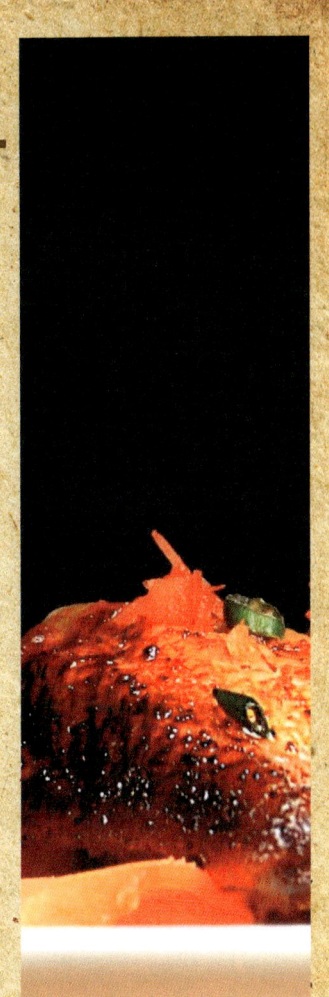

Place the vegetables on a plate and spoon the meatballs on top.

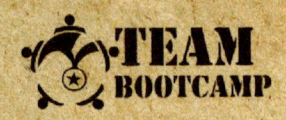

Beef, Butternut Squash & Rosemary Stew

Serves - 4

Cooking time – 90 mins

Prep time – 20 mins

INGREDIENTS:

- Peel and dice the butternut squash into 1 cm pieces.
- Chop the onion and carrot into 1 cm pieces.
- Slice the leek and finely chop the garlic.
- In a large hot pan brown of the beef in the olive oil.
- Add the onion, garlic, carrots, leeks and butternut squash.
- Add the tomato puree, stock and 3 sprigs of rosemary and simmer for 80 minutes.
- Once ready season with the black pepper to taste and serve.

- 500 g diced beef
- 1 butternut squash
- 3 onions
- 1 leek
- Bunch rosemary
- 750 mL beef stock
- 2 carrots
- 1 tsp. olive oil
- 1 tbsp. tomato puree
- 3 cloves garlic
- 1/4 teaspoon cracked black pepper

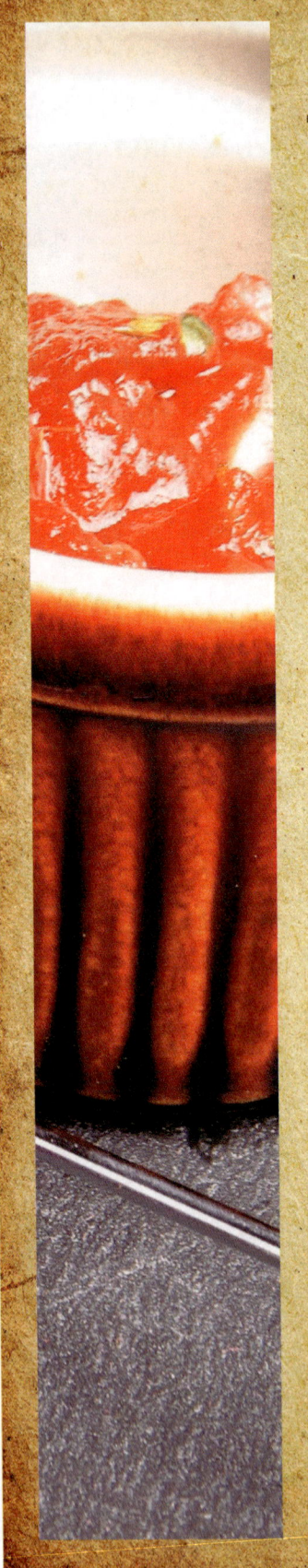

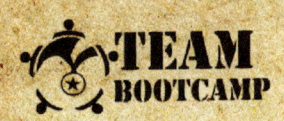

Beef and Spinach Chilli & Mexican Cauliflower Rice

Serves - 4
Cooking time - 90 mins
Prep time - 50 mins

INGREDIENTS:

- For the chilli - Finely chop the onion and chilli peppers.
- In a large hot pan, brown the diced beef and steak mince.
- Add the onion and chilli peppers, cook for 10 more minutes.
- Add the cumin, paprika, chilli powder and tomato puree and cook for a further 5 minutes.
- Add the passatta and jalapenos, simmer for 60-70 min.
- Add the honey and allow to simmer for a further 10 minutes.
- For the rice - Finely chop or grate the cauliflower.
- Finely dice the peppers and chillis.
- Roughly shred the coriander.
- Place the cauliflower, peppers, chilli and turmeric into an oven dish and drizzle with the olive oil.
- Foil the dish and put in a pre-heated oven at 180°C for 25 min.
- Remove from the oven and sprinkle the coriander and stir.
- To serve put the rice on a plate and spoon the chilli on top, finish with chopped coriander.

Chilli

- 300 g lean steak mince
- 300 g diced beef
- 2 onions
- 50 g chopped jalapenos
- 3 medium chilli peppers
- 1 tbsp. cumin
- 1 tbsp. paprika
- 1 tsp. mild chilli powder
- 1 tsp. honey
- 125 g tomato puree
- 400 mL passatta

Rice

- 2 cauliflower
- 150 g finely diced peppers
- Bunch coriander
- 2 medium chillies
- 1/2 teaspoon turmeric
- 1 teaspoon olive oil

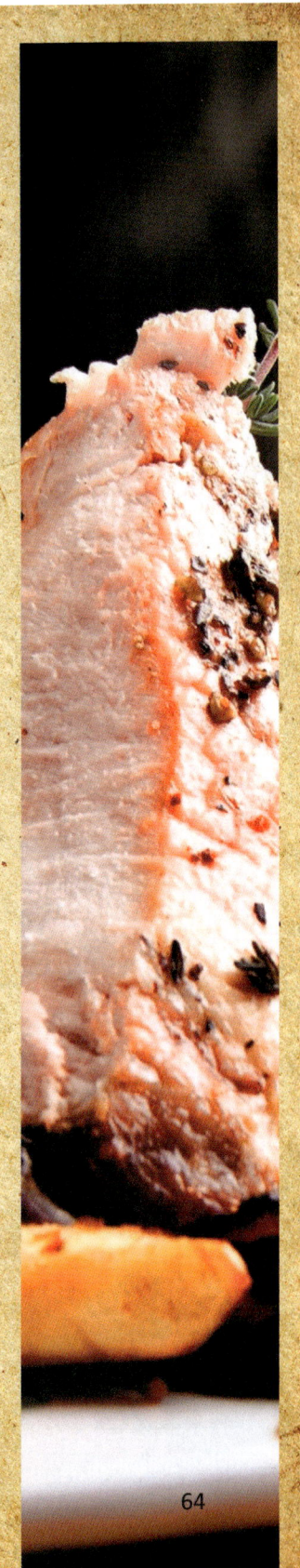

TEAM BOOTCAMP

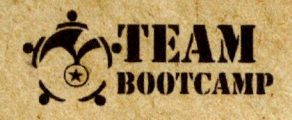

Beef, Butternut Squash & Rosemary Stew

Serves - 4

Cooking time – 80 mins

Prep time – 45 mins

INGREDIENTS:

- Using a tenderizer or rolling pin, put the steaks between 2 sheets of cling film as bash out until 3-4 mm thin.
- Finely dice the onion, garlic and finely slice the mushroom.
- In a hot pan sweat of the onions, mushrooms and garlic.
- To the mix add the mustard, a few thyme leaves, pinch black pepper and a little chopped parsley.
- Stir on a low heat for 5 min and remove from heat and allow to cool.
- Peel and roughly chop the sweet potato and boil for 25 min until soft.
- Lay out the steaks and place the mushroom mix on evenly over the 4 and wrap the steaks around.
- In a very hot pan seal of the olives and put in the oven and 180°C for 35 min
- Top and tail the leeks and in a hot pan fry for 2-3 min and oven for 12 minutes at 180°C

- 4 x 4 oz. rump steaks
- 2 onions
- 4 large flat mushrooms
- Thyme
- 1 tbsp. french mustard
- 12 baby leeks
- 3 sweet potatoes
- 3 cloves garlic
- Parsley
- 1 tbsp. olive oil
- 1/2 tsp. ground black pepper
- Pinch salt
- 800 mL beef stock
- 1 tsp. tomato puree
- 1 tsp. arrowroot

TEAM BOOTCAMP

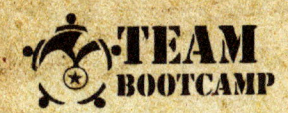

Beef Olives, Braised Baby Leeks & Sweet Potato Puree

Serves - 4

Cooking time - 80 mins

Prep time - 45 mins

INGREDIENTS:

- Using a tenderizer or rolling pin, put the steaks between 2 sheets of cling film as bash out until 3-4 mm thin.
- Finely dice the onion, garlic and finely slice the mushroom.
- In a hot pan sweat of the onions, mushrooms and garlic.
- To the mix add the mustard, a few thyme leaves, pinch black pepper and a little chopped parsley.
- Stir on a low heat for 5 min and remove from heat and allow to cool.
- Peel and roughly chop the sweet potato and boil for 25 min until soft.
- Lay out the steaks and place the mushroom mix on evenly over the 4 and wrap the steaks around.
- In a very hot pan seal of the olives and put in the oven and 180°C for 35 min
- Top and tail the leeks and in a hot pan fry for 2-3 min and oven for 12 minutes at 180°C

- 4 x 4 oz rump steaks
- 2 onions
- 4 large flat mushrooms
- Thyme
- 1 tbsp french mustard
- 12 baby leeks
- 3 sweet potatoes
- 3 cloves garlic
- Parsley
- 1 tbsp olive oil
- 1/2 tsp ground black pepper
- Pinch salt
- 800 mL beef stock
- 1 tsp tomato puree
- 1 tsp arrowroot

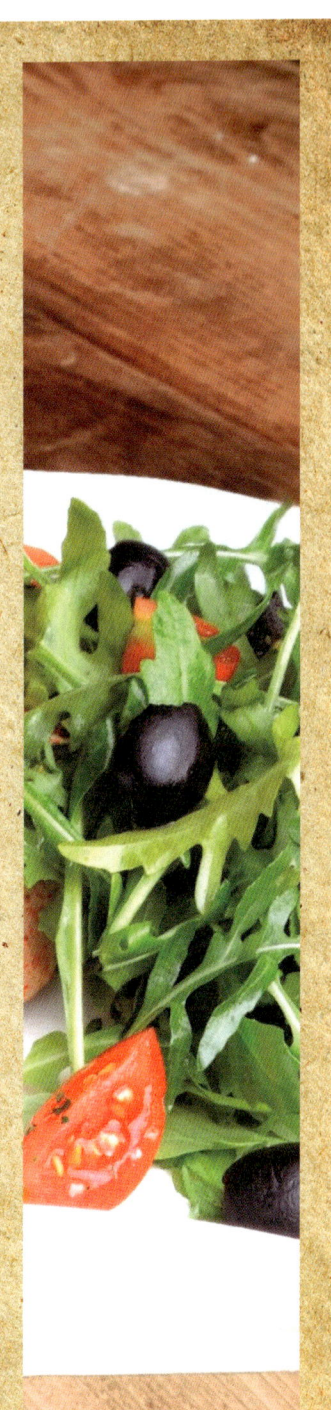

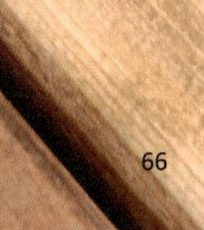

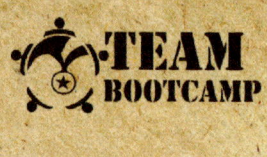

Cottage Pie Topped with Sweat Potato Mash

Serves - 4

Cooking time – 45 mins

Prep time – 15 mins

INGREDIENTS:

- Finely dice the onion and sweat off until soft and allow to cool.
- Finally chop the garlic and chives.
- Finely chop and wash the leeks
- Peel and roughly chop the sweet potato and boil for 20 min
- Using a hot large pan sweat of the onions and leeks, then add the carrots and mince
- Add the tomato puree, thyme and beef stock and simmer for 20 min
- Season to taste with black pepper
- Put in an oven-proof dish and leave for 15-20 minutes
- Drain and mash the sweet potato and neatly place on top of the mince filling, if you have a piping bag and nozzle pipe instead for a neater finish
- Put in a hot oven at 200 º C for 15 min then serve

- 400 g lean steak mince
- 1 large onion
- 2 carrots
- 1 leek
- 3 sweet potatoes
- 1 tbsp tomato puree
- Thyme
- 400 mL beef stock
- Cracked black pepper

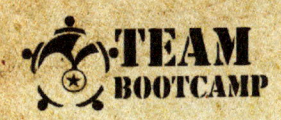

Slow Cooked Brisket with Roasted Veg & Almond Herb Dumplings

Serves - 4

Cooking time - 180 mins

Prep time – 60 mins

INGREDIENTS:

Brisket

- 800 g brisket
- 2 onions
- 4 carrots
- 2 clove garlic
- 1 ltr beef stock
- 1 tsp tomato puree
- Rosemary
- 2 courgettes
- 2 red onions
- 1 butternut squash
- Thyme
- 1 tbsp olive oil

Almond Herb Dumplings

- 125 g arrowroot
- 300 g ground almonds
- Thyme
- Parsley
- 1 tbsp olive oil
- 1 egg
- 2 tbsp cold water
- Pinch cracked black pepper
- Pinch sea salt

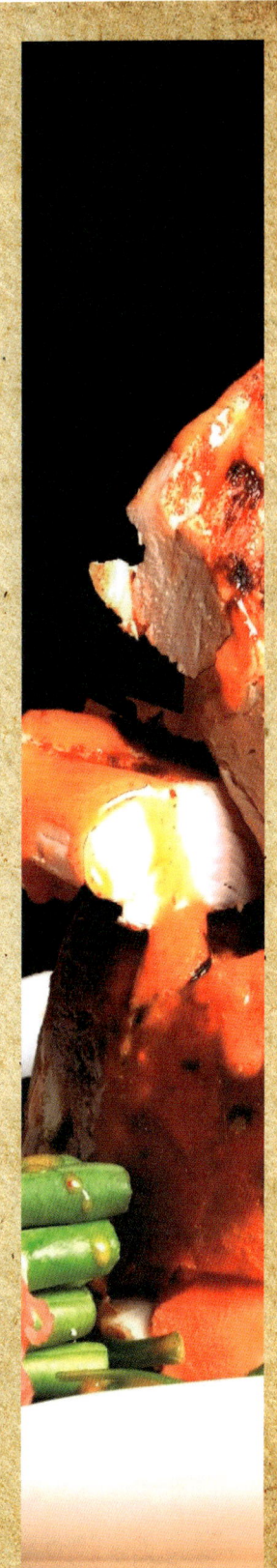

- For the dumplings - Place the arrowroot, almonds, thyme, chopped parsley, olive oil, egg, water, salt and pepper into a bowl and mix until a sticky dough. Roll into 8 small balls and rest in the fridge.
- For the brisket - Roughly chop the onions, carrots and garlic. Using a hot pan brown the brisket and put in an oven dish.
- Brown the onions, carrots and garlic and place into the oven dish over the brisket. Add a few sprigs of thyme.
- Using the same pan again add some of the stock to deglaze the pan and mix in the tomato puree, pour over the brisket. Cover with foil and put in the oven for 120 minutes at 190ºC
- For the roasted vegetables - Peel and cut the butternut squash into 1 cm pieces, chop the red onion and courgettes.
- Coat the vegetables in the olive oil and add a few sprigs of rosemary and toss, put in the oven for 30-40 min at 190ºC.
- Remove the foil from brisket and place dumplings on top, cover again and return to the oven for a further 30 min before serving with the roasted vegetables.

NEW FOR 2015

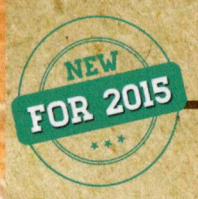

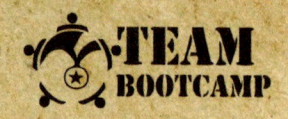

TEAM BOOTCAMP

Beef burger

Serves - 4
Cooking time – 20 mins
Prep time – 20 mins

INGREDIENTS:

- 200g lean beef mince
- 1 onion
- 1 tsp paprika
- 1 tsp mustard
- 1 clove of garlic
- 1 tsp tomato puree
- Small bunch of chives
- Pinch of cracked black pepper

To serve
Paleo salsa
Paleo burger bun

- Finely dice the onion and sweat off until soft and allow to cool.
- Finally chop the garlic and chives.
- Mix the mince, onion, paprika, mustard garlic, tomato puree, chives and black pepper in a bowl until evenly mixed.
- Form the mixture into evenly sized balls and press into burgers. For best results allow to rest for a few hours.
- Heat a griddle pan until very hot and cook the burgers. You may need to finish thicker burgers in the oven to ensure they are cooked thoroughly.
- Serve with a salad and the salsa and paleo bun recipes available in this book.

TEAM BOOTCAMP

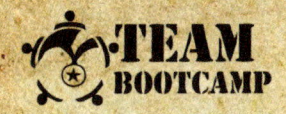

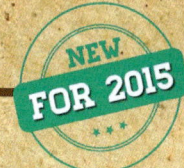

NEW FOR 2015

Sirloin Steak with mushroom and plum tomato

Serves - 2

Cooking time - 15 mins

Prep time - 5 mins

INGREDIENTS:

- Heat 1 tsp of olive oil in a hot pan.
- Slice the shallot and crush the garlic keeping it in one piece.
- In the pan fry the mushrooms then add the shallots and cook for 3 mins.
- Add the tomatoes and a lot of thyme leaves, a pinch of black pepper and garlic clove.
- Place in an oven at 170°c for 4 mins.
- Rub the steaks with the remainder of the oil and a pinch of black pepper and cook on a hot griddle pan for 4 mins either side and allow to rest for 5 mins.
- Serve on the tomatoes, mushrooms and shallots.
- Can be served with sweet potato wedges and side salad.

- 2 6-8oz sirloin steaks
- 1 large shallot
- 2 plum tomatoes
- 4 large flat mushrooms
- Small bunch of thyme
- 2 tsp olive oil
- Cracked black pepper
- 1 clove of garlic

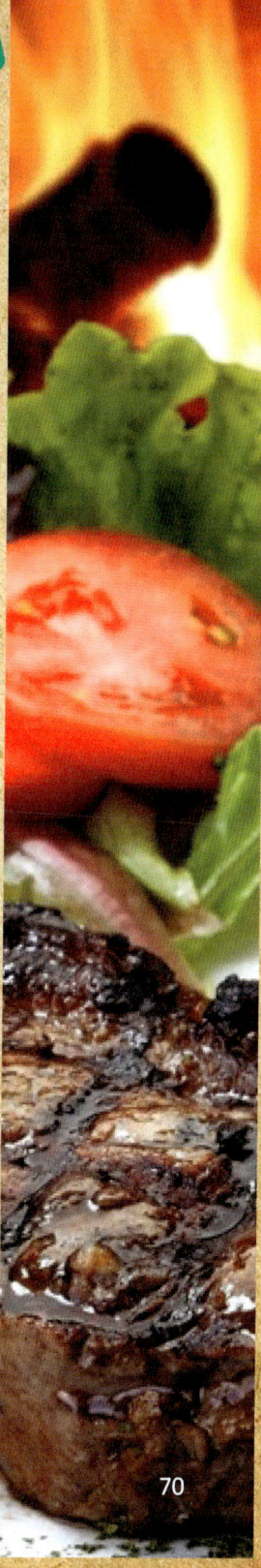

Seafood

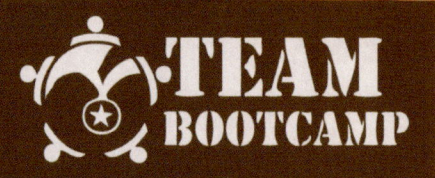

TEAM BOOTCAMP

Salmon Fillet on a Salmon Enfused Medley of Fennel, Asparagus & Roasted Baby Plum Tomatoes

Serves - 4

Cooking time - 30 mins

Prep time – 20 mins

INGREDIENTS:

- Finely chop the parsley and chives.
- Drizzle the tomatoes with 1/2 tsp olive oil and season with a pinch of salt and pepper.
- Slice the fennel and trim the bottoms of asparagus and half them.
- In a hot non-stick pan heat 1/2 tsp olive oil and put the salmon in skin down and put in the oven at 180 ºC for 12 min and rest for 5 min.
- In a hot non-stick pan heat 1 tsp oil and put in the fennel and tomatoes stirring throughout for 3-4 min.
- Add the asparagus, safron, chives and juice of 1/2 lemon.
- Finish with the rocket and take off the heat, season with a pinch of salt and pepper and serve.
- Put on the vegetable mix and the salmon skin side up as it should be crispy.
- Garnish with chopped parsley.

- 4 medium sized salmon fillets
- 2 large whole fennel
- 12 asparagus spears
- 400 g baby plum tomatoes
- 60 g rocket
- Bunch parsley
- Bunch chives
- Cracked black pepper
- Pinch sea salt
- Pinch saffron
- 2 tbsp olive oil

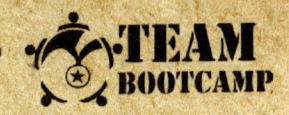

Grilled Whole Plaice, Parmentier Sweet Potato, Pan Fried Kale and a Caper Lemon Sauce

Serves - 4

Cooking time – 30 mins

Prep time – 35 mins

INGREDIENTS:

- Peel and dice the sweet potato into 1 cm pieces and fry off in 1 tsp olive oil, chopped chives, juice of 1/2 lemon, pinch of salt and pepper
- Put in the oven at 180 °C for 30 min.
- Heat a non-stick pan with 1 tsp olive oil and put in the plaice then into the oven at 180 °C for 20 min, seasoned with black pepper and sea salt.
- Finely dice the onion, garlic and parsley.
- Slice the kale and pan fry in 1 tsp olive oil, pinch salt and pepper and let rest when cooked.
- For the sauce use a metal or glass bowl over a Bain Marie and whisk the yolk, vinegar, lemon juice and capers together, add the olive oil while whisking and remove from heat.
- Sweat of the onions and garlic and add the sauce remove from heat and add parsley.
- To serve put on the kale and potato with the plaice on top, pour over the sauce.

- 4 whole plaice
- 2 sweet potatoes
- 1 large kale
- 2 tbsp capers
- 1 lemon
- Bunch chives
- Bunch parsley
- 5 tbsp olive oil
- 1 egg yolk
- 1 tbsp white wine vinegar
- Cracked black pepper
- Pinch sea salt
- 1 small onion
- 1 clove garlic

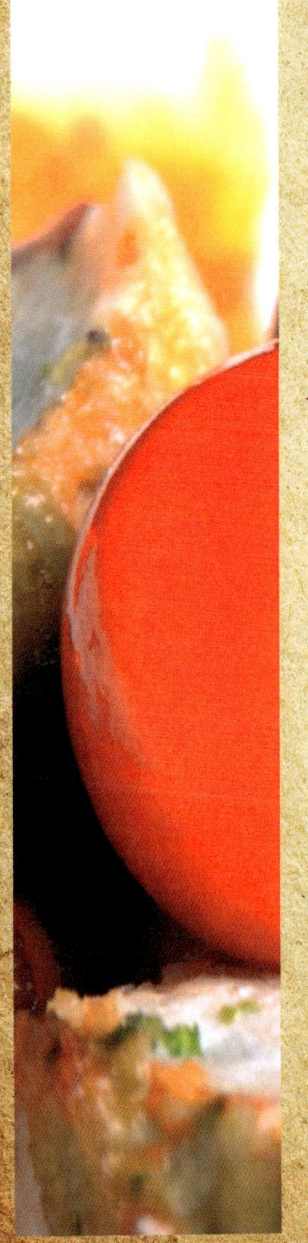

TEAM BOOTCAMP

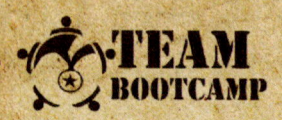

Black Pepper & Almond Calamari with a Chilli & Lime Dip

Serves - 4 Portions

Cooking time - 10 mins

Prep time – 35 mins

INGREDIENTS:

- Cut the squid into rings.
- In 3 dishes put the arrowroot, 1 egg and almonds separate.
- Add the peppers to the almonds.
- Coat the squid in arrowroot then egg then almonds, put on a tray and chill for 1 hour.
- Finely chop the chilli peppers and add to yoghurt.
- Zest and juice the lime and add to yoghurt.
- Season the yoghurt with a pinch of salt and pepper.
- Heat up the oil and fry the squid for no more than 90 seconds.
- Place on a tray when cooked and season with a pinch of salt.
- Serve with the dip and can be served with side salad.

- 2 large squid tubes
- 60 g arrowroot
- 1 egg
- 125 g ground almonds
- 2 small chilli peppers
- 1 lime
- 50 g goat's yoghurt
- Cracked black pepper
- Pinch salt
- 50 mL olive oil

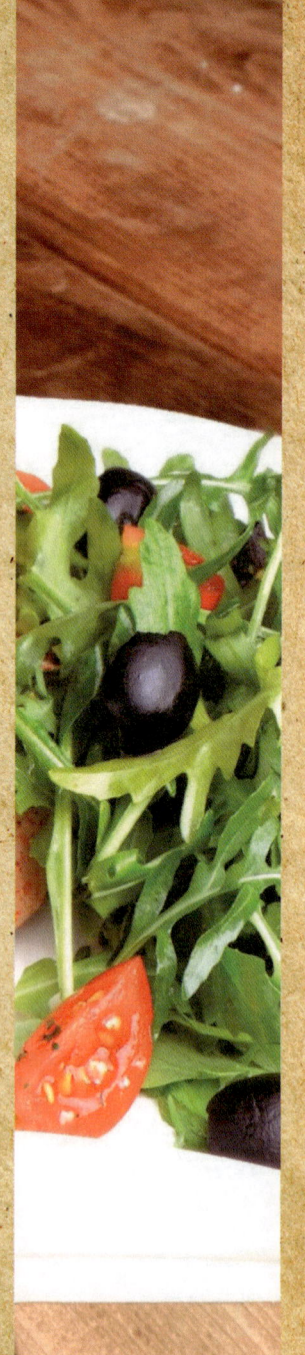

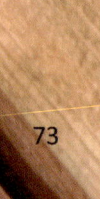

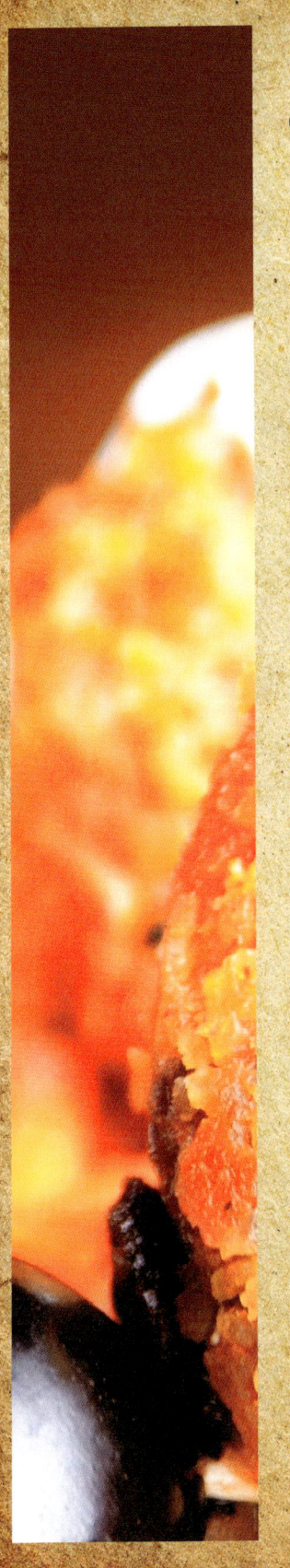

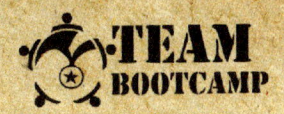

Garlic & Chive Tiger Prawns, Savoy Cabbage Noodles & Cucumber & Horseradish Pickle

Serves - 4

Cooking time - 15 mins

Prep time - 25 mins

INGREDIENTS:

- 600 g tiger prawns
- 2 cloves garlic
- Bunch chives
- 1 lemon
- 1 tsp white wine
- 1 large savoy cabbage
- 3 tbsp olive oil
- 1/2 cucumber
- 1/2 fresh horseradish
- 50 mL white wine vinegar
- 1/2 tsp fennel seeds
- 1/2 tsp mustard seeds
- 4 cardamom pods
- 1 mild chilli pepper
- Cracked black pepper
- Pinch salt

- Finely strip the horseradish and cucumber and add to the vinegar, fennel seed, and cardamom pods in a dish.
- Finely chop the chilli pepper and add to the mix with a pinch of salt and pepper.
- Finely slice the cabbage.
- Finely chop the chives and garlic.
- Heat a pan with 2 tsp oil and put in the prawns, stir for 3-5 min.
- Add the garlic and stir for 2 min.
- Add the juice from 1/2 lemon and the wine stir for 2 more min and remove from heat to sit for 4-5 min.
- In another hot pan heat the last of the oil and fry the cabbage, season with a pinch of salt and pepper.
- To serve put the cabbage on the plate and prawns on top, drizzle with the sauce left in the pan and serve the pickle in a dish on the side.

TEAM BOOTCAMP

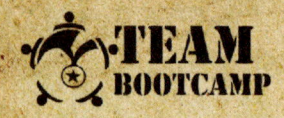

Paleo Fish, Chips & Tartar Sauce

Serves - 4 Portions

Cooking time - 45 mins

Prep time – 40 mins

INGREDIENTS:

- First cut the sweet potatoes into chips, toss in a little oil, season well and put on an oven tray in the oven at 180°C for 35 min.
- In 3 dishes put the arrowroot, 2 egg beaten and almonds separately.
- Season the arrowroot with a pinch of salt and pepper and add the fish fillet, then to the egg mix and finally almonds ensuring evenly coated and chill in fridge for 10-15 min.
- For the tartar sauce, blend the yolk of 3 eggs, Dijon, juice of 1/2 lemon, caper, girkin, wine, 65 ml olive oil and pinch of salt and pepper.
- Finish the sauce with some chopped parsley and chill.
- Heat the last of the oil and fry the fish for 3 min each side and finish in the oven a 180°C for 10 min then serve with the chips and sauce.

- 4 small haddock, cod or Pollock fillets
- 5 eggs
- 75 g arrowroot
- 250 g ground almonds
- 75 mL olive oil
- 2 large sweet potatoes
- 1 girkin
- 1 tsp baby capers or chopped capers
- 1 lemon
- 1 tsp Dijon mustard
- 50 mL white wine
- Cracked black pepper
- Sea salt
- Bunch parsley

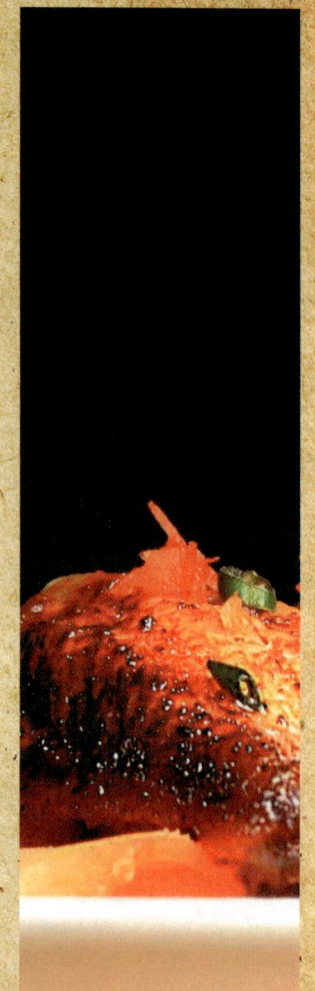

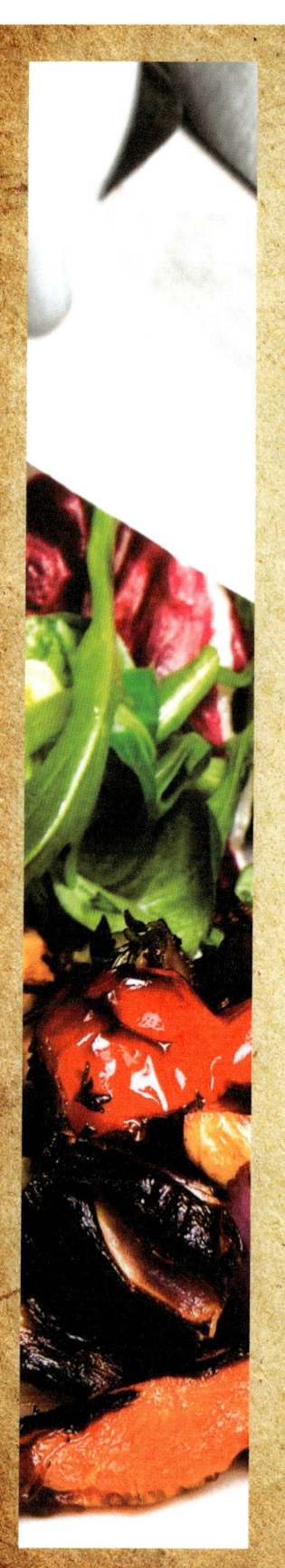

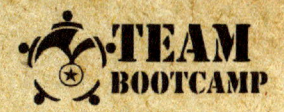

Smoked Haddock on Wilted Spinach with Celeriac Chips & Poached Egg

Serves - 4 Portions

Cooking time – 40 mins

Prep time – 20 mins

INGREDIENTS:

- First peel and cut the celeriac into chunky chips and seal in a pan with 1 tsp oil, season well and put in the oven at 190 ºC for 30 min.
- Heat up a pan and with the oil place in the haddock and season with pepper, place the spinach around and put in the oven at 190 ºC for 8-10 min.
- Get a deep pan at hot water with a tsp white wine vinegar, ensuring its hot but not boiling, poach the eggs for 4-5 min.
- To serve stack the chips with the haddock on top and the egg on top of that, place the spinach around and finish with cracked black pepper over the egg.

- 1 tsp white wine vinegar
- 4 portions smoked haddock
- 80 g spinach
- 2 medium celeriac
- 4 eggs
- 2 tbsp olive oil
- Bunch dill
- Cracked black pepper
- Sea salt

TEAM BOOTCAMP

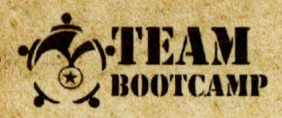

Baked Trout in Lemon & Parsley with Pan Seared Shredded Vegetables

Serves - 4 Portions

Cooking time - 30 mins

Prep time – 25 mins

INGREDIENTS:

- Using baking parchment wrap the trout individually with a squeeze of half a lemon on each and season well with salt and pepper.
- Put in the oven at 200ºC for 15-17 min then allow to rest.
- Finely strip the carrots, leek, and fennel and chop the parsley.
- Using a hot pan, heat the oil and add the carrots and fennel.
- Cook for 2 min then add the leek, pak choi and season with a pinch of salt and pepper.
- To serve place the fish on a plate covering the paper and placing the vegetables on top.
- Finish with chopped parsley and serve.

- 4 whole small trout
- 2 lemon
- Bunch parsley
- 2 carrots
- 1 leek
- 1 fennel
- 1 pak choi
- 1 tbsp olive oil
- Cracked black pepper
- Sea salt

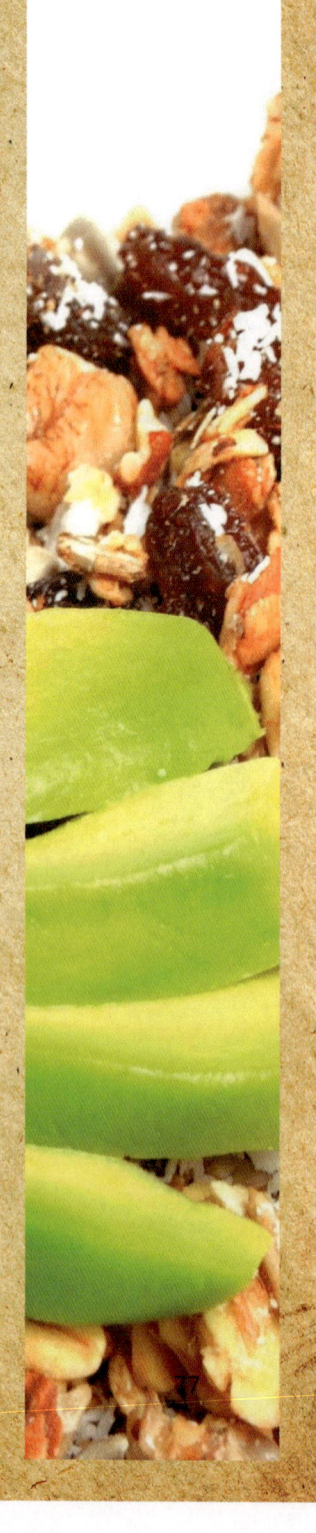

Chicken

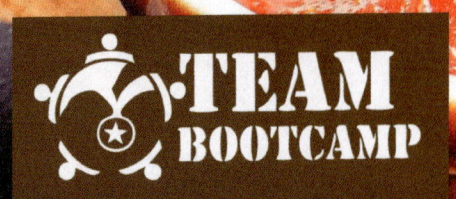

Chicken & Vegetable Skewers with Spiced Rice

Serves - 6

Cooking time – 35 mins

Prep time - 45 mins

INGREDIENTS:

- Dice the chicken, courgette, onion and pepper into large chunks.
- Finely chop the chilli, garlic and coriander.
- Put the chilli, garlic, coriander, fennel seeds, cumin and paprika into a bowl with the olive oil and mix.
- Using 6 large skewers push on chicken, courgettes, onion and peppers until it is all on the skewers.
- Using a large flat oven tray, put the chicken skewers on ensuring they're not touching and with a spoon, drizzle the spice and oil mix over them until they're evenly covered.
- Cover with cling film and allow to marinade for 1-2 hrs if possible.
- For the rice, finely chop or grate the cauliflower, finely chop the chilli and onion.
- Using an oven proof dish ass the cauliflower, oil, chilli, turmeric, garam masala, onion and bay leaves, mix thoroughly and cover with foil.
- Heat the oven to 200°C and cook chicken for 20 min.
- Place the rice in the oven for 15 min and serve.

Skewers

- 1 tsp olive oil
- 3 chicken breasts
- 1 courgette
- 2 red onions
- 2 red peppers
- 1 medium chilli
- 1/2 teaspoon fennel seeds
- 1/2 teaspoon ground cumin
- 1/2 teaspoon paprika
- 1 clove garlic coriander

Rice

- 1 tsp olive oil
- 2 cauliflowers
- 1 medium chilli
- 1 teaspoon turmeric
- 1/2 teaspoon garam masala
- 1 small onion
- 2 bay leaves

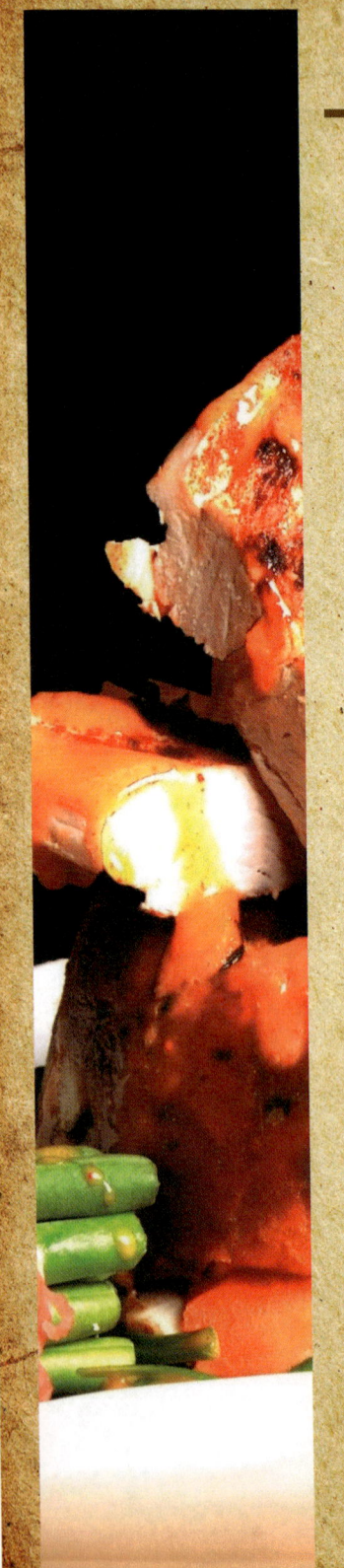

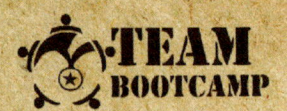

Chicken & Chorizo Salad

Serves - 6

Cooking time – 20 mins

Prep time – 30 mins

INGREDIENTS:

- Slice the chicken into thin strips.
- Finely strip the carrot, cucumber and spring onions.
- Quarter the tomato taking out the seeds and then finely strip.
- Using a very hot non-stick pan brown off the chicken.
- Add the chorizo to the pan and continue to cook for 5-8 min and allow to rest for 3-4 min.
- Using a large bowl place the mixed leaves, tomatoes, carrot, cucumber, spring onion and olive oil and toss.
- In 6 serving bowls place the salad mix in a spoon on top the chicken and chorizo mix.
- Finish the dish with a squeeze of lime and serve.

- 3 chicken breasts
- 250 g chopped chorizo
- 1 lime
- Basil
- 200 g mixed leaves
- 3 tomatoes
- 1 carrot
- 1/2 cucumber
- 4 spring onions
- 1 tbsp extra virgin olive oil

TEAM BOOTCAMP

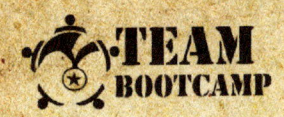

Chicken & Butternut Squash Bake

Serves – 4

Cooking time – 45 mins

Prep time – 40 mins

INGREDIENTS:

- Peel and dice the butternut squash.
- Dice the chicken, onion and slice the leek.
- Finely chop the garlic and parsley.
- In a hot pan brown off the chicken and then add the butternut squash, onion, leeks and garlic and continue to cook.
- Add the chicken stock and 2 sprigs of thyme and simmer for 10 min.
- Season with salt and pepper to taste and pour into an oven-proof dish.
- Top with flaked almonds and cook in the oven at 160°C for 25 min ensuring the almonds don't brown.
- Finish the dish with some chopped parsley and serve.

- 2 chicken breasts
- 1 butternut squash
- 1 onion
- 1 leek
- 2 cloves garlic
- 300 ml chicken stock
- Thyme
- Parsley
- 50 g flaked almonds
- Cracked black pepper
- Pinch sea salt

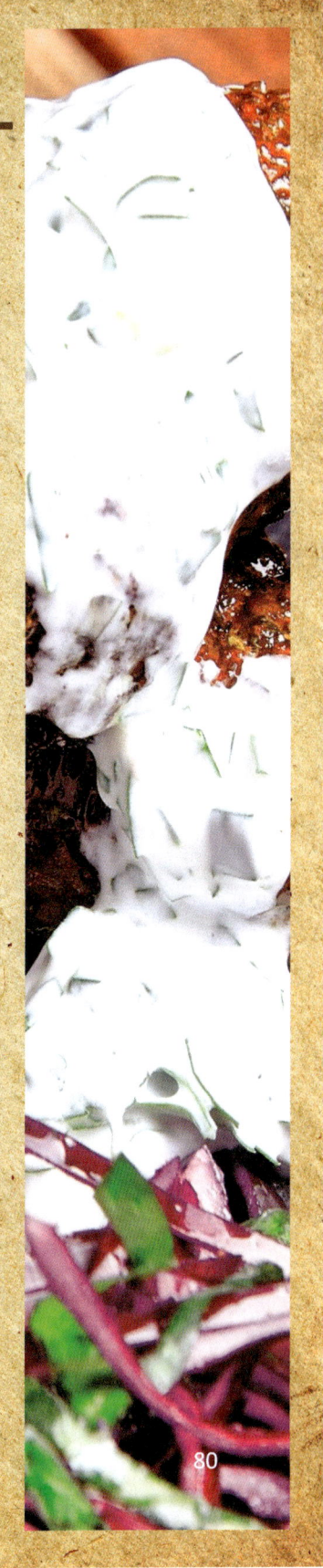

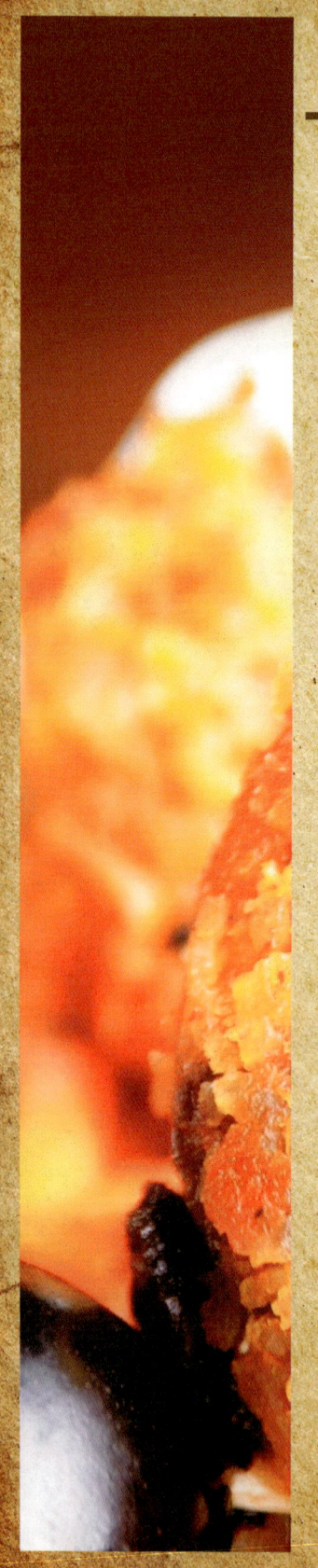

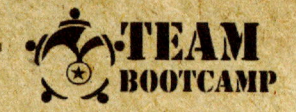

Pesto Chicken on Sweet Potato, Fennel & Roast Tomatoes

Serves - 4

Cooking time – 60 mins

Prep time – 50 mins

- For the pesto, using a blender add the basil leaves, garlic, olive oil and pine nuts. Blend until smooth.
- Season the mix with salt and pepper to taste.
- Peel the sweet potato and dice into 1 cm pieces.
- Slice the fennel and garlic.
- Quarter the tomatoes.
- In a hot pan warm the olive oil and put in the sweet potato, fennel and garlic and toss for 2-3 min season with pepper.
- Place the mix into a large oven tray and add the tomatoes.
- Using a hot oven-proof pan seal of the chicken and coat in the pesto and put in the oven at 180ºC for 20 minutes.
- Put the veg in the oven at 180ºC for 15 min.
- Once done mix the rocket through the roast veg and then serve with the chicken breast on top.

INGREDIENTS:

Pesto

- 1 bunch basil
- 2 cloves garlic
- 150 mL olive oil
- 100 g pinenuts
- Pinch ground black pepper
- Pinch salt

Chicken and Vegetables

- 4 small chicken breasts
- 2 sweet potatoes
- 2 cloves garlic
- 2 whole fennel
- 4 plum tomatoes
- 1 lemon
- 30 g rocket
- Cracked black pepper
- 1 tsp olive oil

TEAM BOOTCAMP

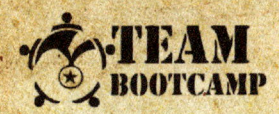

Feta & Spinach Stuff Chicken with Radish and Beetroot Salad

Serves - 4

Cooking time – 25 mins

Prep time – 30 mins

INGREDIENTS:

- Butterfly chicken breasts.
- Chop or crumble feta and mix with spinach and pinch black pepper.
- Stuff the chicken with feta mix and ensure there are no gaps when thicken is wrapped around filling.
- Season the breasts.
- Heat up a pan until very hot with the oil and seal the chicken for 2 min either side and place in an oven at 200ºC for 18 min.
- Remove and allow to rest for 5 min.
- Slice the radish and beetroot into disks and add to salad leaves.
- Zest 1/4 lemon and add to salad mix.
- Put salad in a bowl and place chicken on top, you can slice if preferred.
- Using half the lemon finish the dish with squeezing the juice over and serve.

- 80 g feta
- 40 g spinach
- 4 small chicken breasts
- 8 salad radish
- 4 small whole beetroot
- 1 lemon
- 100 g salad leaves
- 1/4 tsp cracked black pepper
- 1 tbsp olive oil

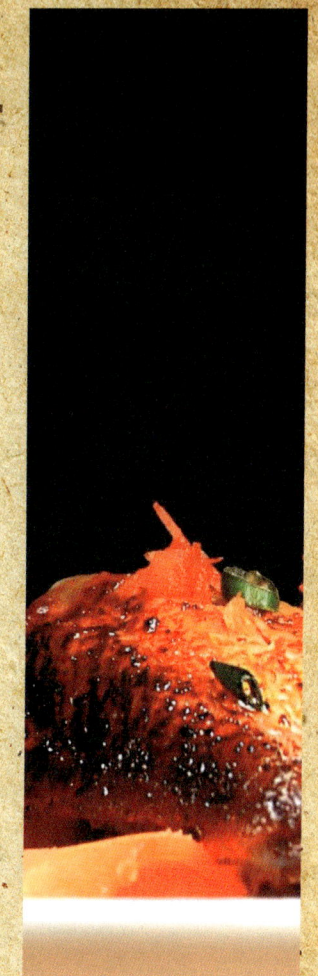

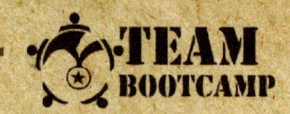

Curried Coconut Chicken & Cauliflower Rice

Serves - 6

Cooking time – 60 mins

Prep time – 40 mins

INGREDIENTS:

Curry

- Dice the chicken, onions and butternut squash into 1 cm pieces.
- Finely chop the garlic and chillis.
- In a hot large pan brown the diced chicken.
- Add the onions, butternut squash and garlic and sweat for 5 min.
- Add the garam masala, cumin, turmeric, paprika, chilli and black pepper and fry off for 5 min.
- Add the chopped tomatoes and simmer for 35 min.
- Finish with the coconut cream and chopped coriander.

Rice

- Finely chop or grate the cauliflower.
- In an oven-proof dish ass cauliflower, oil, coriander, cardamom and black pepper.
- Foil dish and put in over at 190 degrees C for 20 min and serve.

Curry

- 600 g chicken thighs
- 2 onions
- 1 butternut squash
- 2 cloves garlic
- 60 g spinach
- 1 tin coconut cream
- 1 tbsp garam masala
- 1 tbsp cumin
- 1 tbsp turmeric
- 1 tsp paprika
- 4 medium chillis
- Bunch coriander
- 1 tsp cracked black pepper
- 2 tin chopped tomatoes

Rice

- 2 cauliflowers
- 1 tsp olive oil
- Coriander
- 6 cardamom pods
- Cracked black pepper

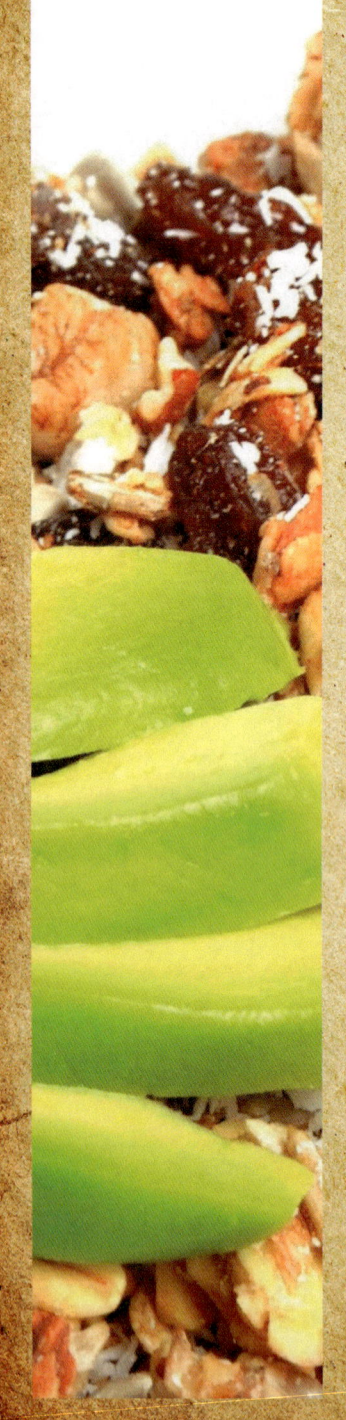

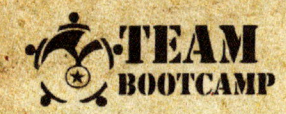

Lemon & Thyme Chicken with Roasted Vegetables

Serves - 4

Cooking time – 40 mins

Prep time – 20 mins

INGREDIENTS:

- Marinate the chicken in the zest of 1 lemon, 2-4 sprigs of thyme, chopped garlic and pinch black pepper.
- Chop the courgettes, red, yellow and green pepper and red onion into 2 cm pieces and place in an oven-proof dish
- Using a very hot pan add a drizzle of olive oil seal off the chicken until golden brown and put in the oven at 170ºC for 20 min.
- Using a very hot pan and remainder of oil, panfry all the chopped veg and then add to the oven at 170ºC for 12 minutes.
- Remove chicken and veg and add some thyme leaves to veg and stir.
- To serve put the veg on a plate and a breast on top squeezing lemon juice over to finish.

- 2 tbsp olive oil
- 1 lemon
- Small bunch thyme
- 1 clove garlic
- 4 small chicken breasts
- 2 courgettes
- 1 red pepper
- 1 yellow pepper
- 1 red onion
- Cracked black pepper
- Pinch sea salt

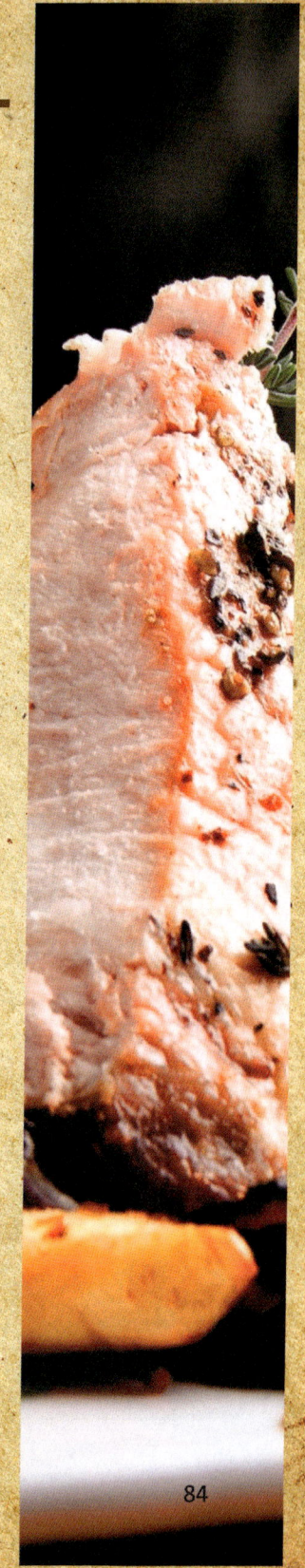

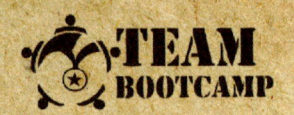

Chicken & Pepper Enchiladas

Serves - 4

Cooking time – 30 mins

Prep time – 60 mins

INGREDIENTS:

- To make the pancake mix all ingredients together, using a hot non-stick pan pour some of the batter in till base of the pan is coated. Once bubbles appear turn and cook on the other side for 30-60 seconds and allow pancakes to cool.
- Slice the chicken, onion, peppers, quarter the tomato and finely chop the chilli.
- Using a hot pan brown off the chicken breast.
- Add the onion, peppers and chilli and cook for 1-2 min.
- Turn down the heat to a medium setting and add the cumin and paprika, cook the mix further for 1-2 min.
- Split the mix evenly onto the pancakes and wrap.
- Put in the oven for 5-8 minutes then serve.
- It can be served with salad, homemade salsa, cauliflower rice or on its own as a lighter meal.

Tortilla/Pancake

- 125 g arrowroot
- 1 egg
- 1 tsp cold water
- Pinch salt

Chicken Filling

- 2 chicken breasts
- 1 onion
- 3 mixed peppers
- 3 tomatoes
- 1 tsp honey
- 1 medium chilli
- 1 tsp ground cumin
- 1 tsp paprika

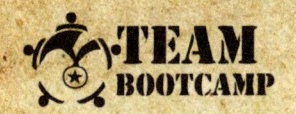

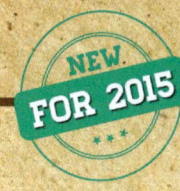

Sesame chicken on stir fry vegetables

Serves - 4

Cooking time – 30 mins

Prep time – 10 mins

INGREDIENTS:

- Finely chop the chilli and garlic.
- Pick the pak choi but leave the leaf intact.
- Slice the red pepper, onion, courgette, spring onion and coriander.
- Heat half the oil and add the chicken to colour both sides.
- Drizzle honey on the chicken and reduce in the pan until very sticky then pour in the sesame seeds coating the chicken evenly.
- Place in an oven at 170°c for 12 mins.
- While the chicken cooks, heat the remainder of the oil in a wok. Add the onions, peppers and spring onions and stir fry for 2 mins.
- Add the chilli, garlic and black pepper and cook for a further 2 min. Remove from the heat and let sit.
- Once cooked serve the vegetables on a plate with the chicken on top. Finish with a squeeze of lime and chopped coriander.

- 4 medium chicken breasts
- 50g sesame seeds
- 20g honey
- Small bunch of coriander
- 1 lime
- 1 green chilli
- 2 cloves of garlic
- 2 pak choi
- 1 red pepper
- 1 red onion
- 1 courgette
- Bunch of spring onions
- 1 tbsp olive oil
- Small pinch of black pepper

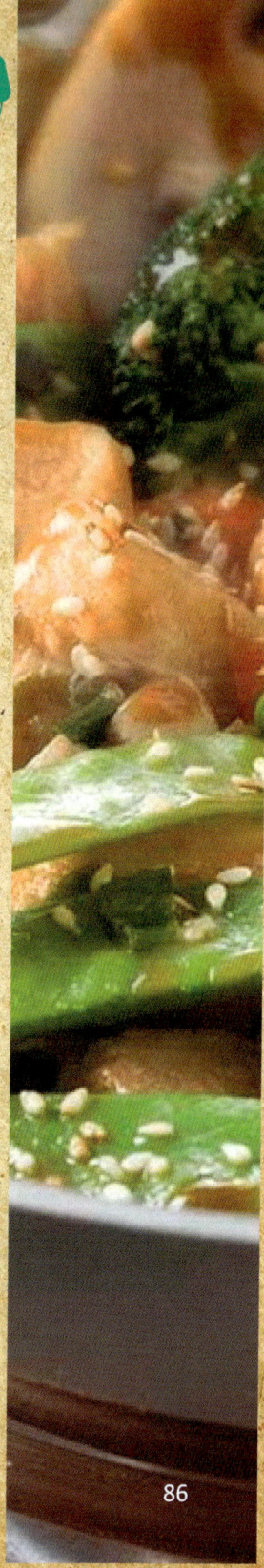

NEW FOR 2015

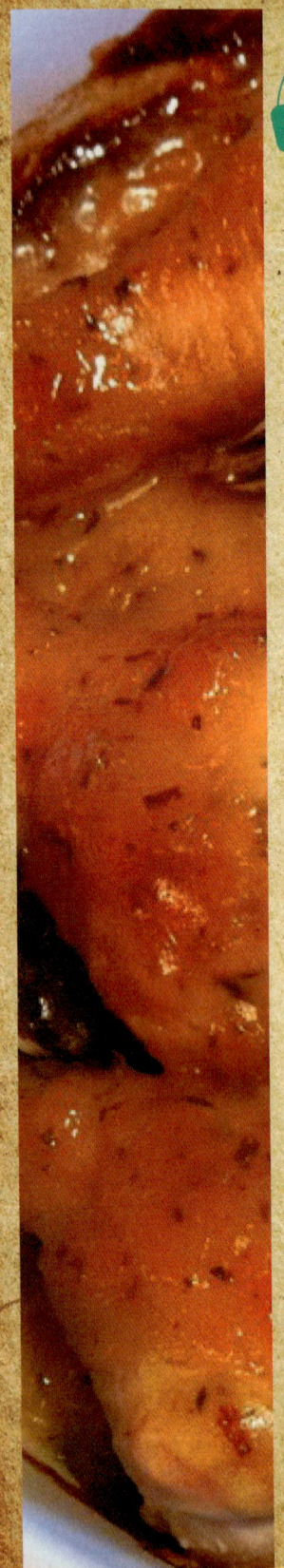

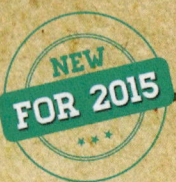

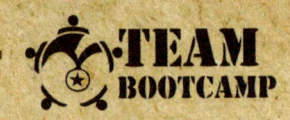

TEAM BOOTCAMP

Honey and Mustard Chicken

Serves - 4

Cooking time – 10 mins

Prep time – 10 mins

INGREDIENTS:

- In a small hot pan heat half the oil and sweat the sliced shallot for 3 mins.
- Add the honey and mustard and simmer for 3-4 mins, remove from the heat and add a pinch of black pepper.
- Heat the remainder of the oil in another pan and seal off the chicken for about 3 mins either side.
- Add the honey and mustard mix to the chicken and ensure the chicken is evenly coated.
- Place in an oven at 200°c for 8 mins.
- Once removed from oven, allow to rest for 3-5 minutes and finish with chopped chives.
- To serve – Slice the chicken and serve with salad or steamed vegetables.

- 4 small chicken breasts
- 1 shallot
- bunch of chives
- 1 tbsp wholegrain mustard
- 1 tbsp honey
- Pinch salt
- Cracked black pepper
- 1 tsp olive oil

Pork

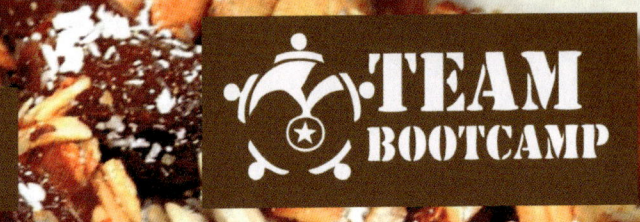

Sage & Onion Sausages

Serves - 6

Cooking time – 25 mins

Prep time – 40 mins

INGREDIENTS:

- Using a food processor place the onions, small handful sage, nutmeg, pinch black pepper and garlic and blend till quite fine but not smooth.
- In a bowl add the mince and mix from the food processor.
- Add a pinch of salt and mix thoroughly.
- Using a piping bag and round long ended nozzle pipe the meat filling into the skins.
- Twist the skins to the desired size of sausage and place in the fridge to rest for 1-2 hours if possible.
- To cook, cut at the twisted area and using a hot no stick pan brown the sausages and finish in the oven.
- Or you can frill then serve.

- 1 pig skin/sausage skin
- 400 g pork mince
- 2 onions
- Sage
- 1/4 tsp nutmeg
- Cracked black pepper
- Pinch salt
- 1 clove garlic

TEAM BOOTCAMP

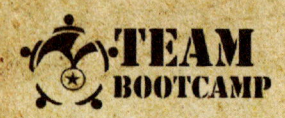

Sweat & Sour Pork with Stir Fried Pak Choi

Serves - 4

Cooking time – 30 mins

Prep time – 40 mins

INGREDIENTS:

- For the sauce - Finely shop the garlic.
- Using a hot pan sweat the garlic and then add the fennel seeds, cinnamon, star anise, black pepper and vinegar and simmer for 5 min.
- Add the tomato puree and honey and cook for a further 3 min.
- Add the chicken stock and simmer for 10 more min.
- Add a tsp cold water to the arrowroot and add to the simmering sauce, cook for 5 more min then pass through a sieve and put to side.
- For the pork - Strip the pork loin.
- Finely slice the onion, red pepper, green pepper and garlic.
- Using a hot wok or large frying pan, brown of the pork then add the garlic and onion, cook for 10 min stirring throughout.
- Add the green and red peppers, pak choi and cook for 5 more min stirring throughout.
- Finish the dish by pouring the sauce over, simmer for 3-5 min then serve.
- It can be served with either cauliflower, rice or squash noodles.

- 400 g pork loin
- 1 red onion
- 1 red pepper
- 1 green pepper
- 2 cloves garlic
- 4 pak choi

Sauce

- 100 g honey
- 100 g tomato puree
- 500 ml white wine vinegar
- 50 ml chicken or vegetable stock
- 1/4 tsp ground black pepper
- 1/4 tsp fennel seeds
- 1/8 tsp cinnamon
- 1 star anise
- 1 clove garlic
- 1 tbsp arrowroot

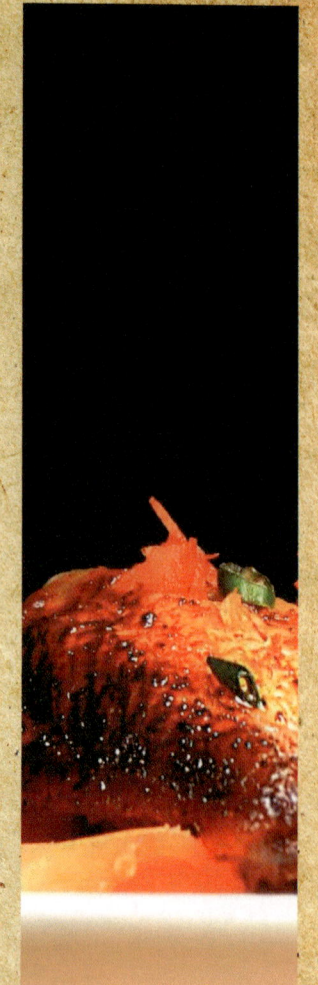

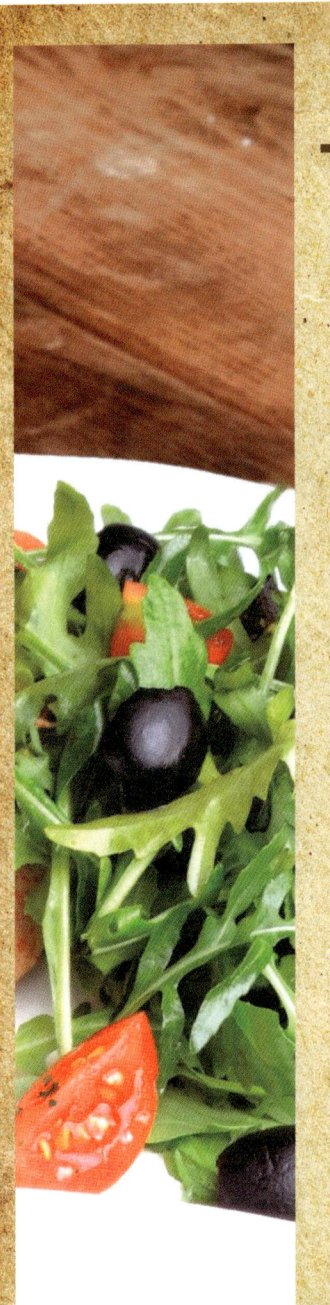

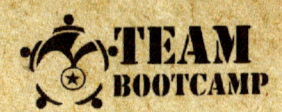

Pork Loin Apple & Shallot Gravy

Serves - 4

Cooking time – 40 mins

Prep time – 30 mins

INGREDIENTS:

- Peel and quarter the shallots.
- Peel and cut the apple into segments.
- Place the shallots, apple and honey in an oven tray and roast for 25 min.
- Roughly chop the garlic and sweat in a hot pan.
- Add the thyme and stock and leave to simmer.
- Season the pork steaks with a pinch of black pepper and salt.
- Using a very hot pan seal the steaks for 3-4 min both sides, place on a tray and finish in the oven for 15 min.
- Remove the stock from the stove and pass through a sieve.
- Remove the shallots and apples from the oven and put the tray directly on the heat adding the stock and stirring.
- Remove steaks from the oven and spoon the shallot and apple gravy over to serve.
- This dish can be served with roasted veg, sweet potato ship or sweet potato mash.

- 4 x 4 oz pork loin steaks
- 3 large shallots
- 1 clove garlic
- 1 large Bramley apple
- 2 sprigs of thyme
- 1 tsp olive oil
- 300 ml pork or vegetable stock
- 1 tsp honey
- Cracked black pepper
- Pinch salt

TEAM BOOTCAMP

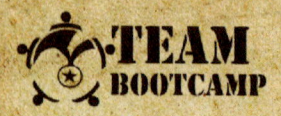

Pork, Thyme & Leek Pie

Serves - 4

Cooking time – 90 mins

Prep time – 40 mins

INGREDIENTS:

- For the pastry, using a mixing bowl add the almonds, arrowroot, olive oil and 1 egg yolk and mix until a dough and put in the fridge to rest.
- For the filling, slice and wash the leeks.
- Finely chop the carrot, onion, sage and garlic.
- Using a hot pan brown the pork in the olive oil.
- Add the carrot, leeks, onion and garlic and cook and stir for 10 min.
- Add the tomato puree and stock and simmer for 20 min.
- Season to taste with salt and pepper, add sage and put in a oven dish.
- Roll out the pastry using a sprinkle of arrowroot so it doesn't stick.
- Put in the oven at 160 °C for 35-45 min then serve.

Pastry
- 400 g ground almonds
- 150 g arrowroot
- 1 egg
- 1 tbsp olive oil

Pie Filling
- 500 g diced pork
- 2 leeks
- 1 onion
- 1 carrot
- Sage
- 1 clove garlic
- 500 g pork or vegetable stock
- 1 tsp olive oil
- 1 tbsp tomato puree
- Pinch cracked black pepper
- Pinch sea salt

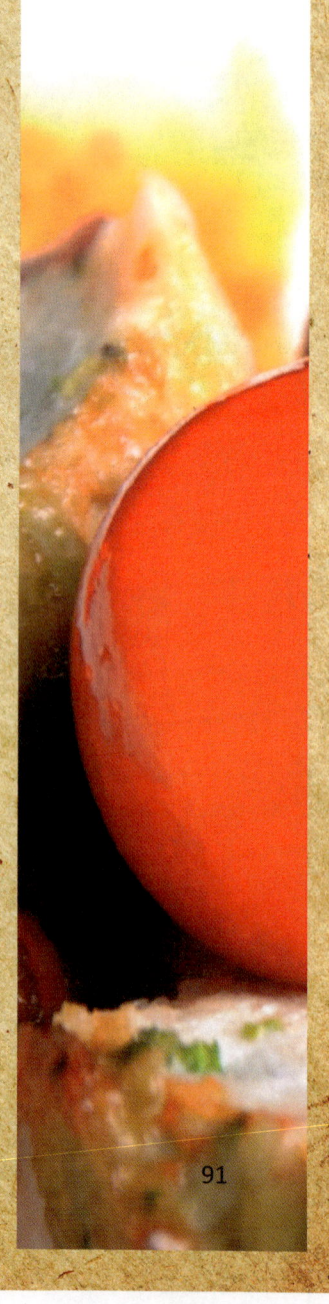

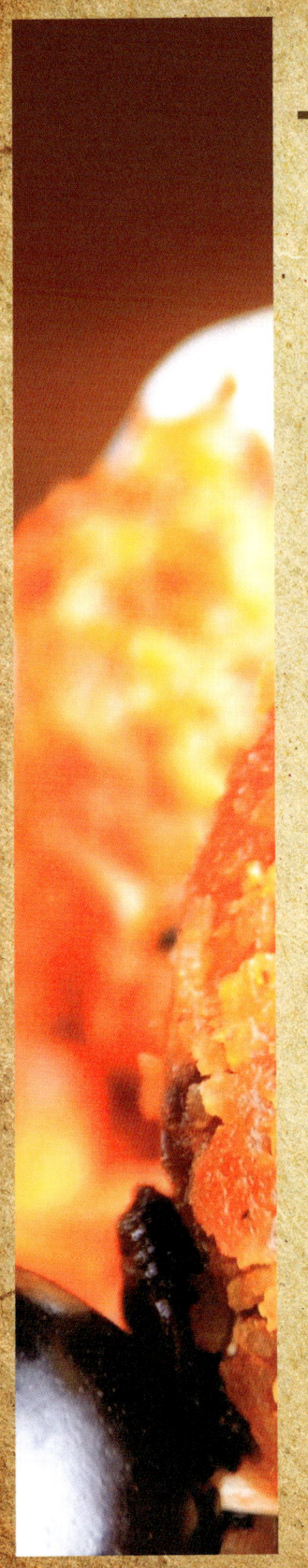

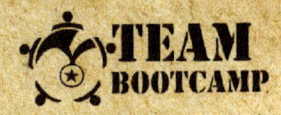

Chilli & Pepper Pork Chop, Sweet Potato Wedges, Roast Peppers & Cherry Tomatoes

Serves - 4

Cooking time – 60 mins

Prep time – 25 mins

INGREDIENTS:

- Finely chop the chilli peppers and chives and put over the pork chops.
- Over the pork pour 1 tbsp oil, add pink peppercorns, pinch black pepper and pinch sea salt and allow to sit in fridge for 15-20 min.
- Wash and cut the sweet potato into wedges put in the oven at 180 ºC for 45 min.
- Roughly cut the red, yellow, and green pepper.
- In a oven tray add the red, yellow and green pepper with the tomatoes, oil, salt and pepper.
- Put in the oven at 180 degrees for 30 min.
- Using a hot pan brown the pork chops and put on an oven tray in the oven at 180 ºC for 18-20 min.
- Serve with torn basil leaves and coriander.

- 4 x 4 - 6 oz pork chops
- 2 sweet potatoes
- 1 red pepper
- 1 yellow pepper
- 1 green pepper
- 12 cherry tomatoes
- 2 medium chilli peppers
- 1 tsp pink peppercorns
- 2 tbsp olive oil
- Cracked black pepper
- Chives
- Basil
- Sea salt

TEAM BOOTCAMP

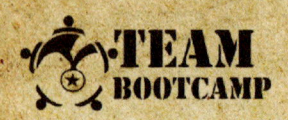

BBQ Ribs

Serves - 6

Cooking time – 120 mins

Prep time – 40 mins

INGREDIENTS:

- To start put the ribs in a deep oven tray and pour 1 litre of stock over, foil and put in the oven at 190 °C for 100 min.
- For the sauce finely chop the onion, garlic and tomatoes.
- Sweat of the onion and garlic in a large pot.
- Add the vinegar and simmer for 10 min.
- Add the tomato puree, tomatoes, stock, celery, salt, Worcestershire sauce, passatta, mustard, black pepper, bay leaves and honey and simmer for 30 min.
- Remove bay leaves and blend sauce till smooth no need to sieve.
- Once ribs are cooled so that they are soft, place on another tray to dry for 3-4 min then cut to desired size.
- Coat in the sauce and put in the oven at 220 °C for 15-20 min then serve.

- 2-3 racks pork ribs
- 1.5 ltr vegetable stock
- 10 tomatoes
- 200 g tomato puree
- 1 onion
- 2 cloves garlic
- 1/2 teaspoon celery salt
- 3-4 tablespoons Worcestershire sauce
- 400 ml passatta
- 2 tsp English mustard
- 1 tbsp black pepper
- 220 g honey
- 2 bay leaves
- 60 ml white wine vinegar

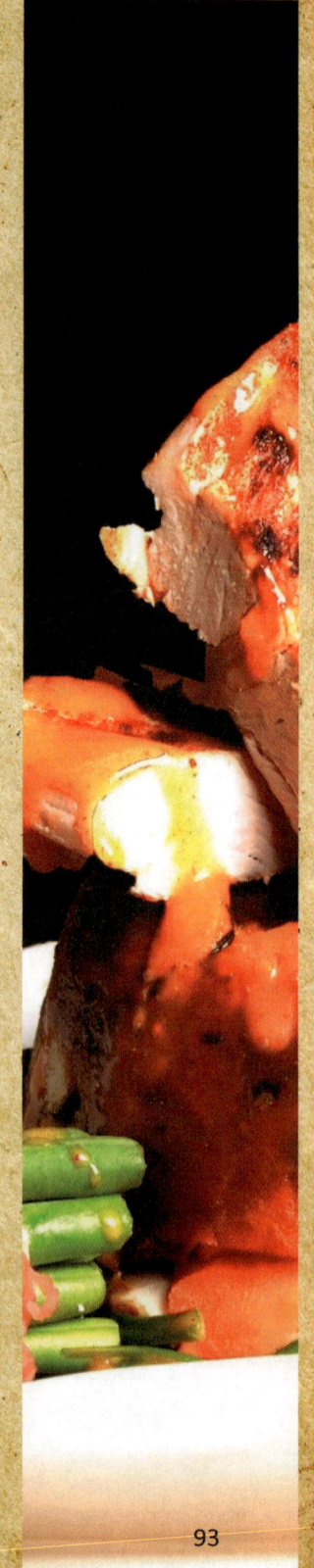

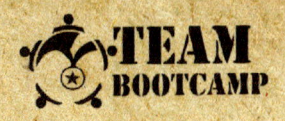

Pulled Pork with Fennel, Asparagus & Tomato Medley

Serves – 4

Cooking time – 120 mins

Prep time – 30 mins

INGREDIENTS:

- Using a large hot pan, brown the whole leg in the olive oil.
- Add the stock, black peppercorns, bay leaves and sage
- Cut the garlic bulb in half and add to pan and cook for 120 min on a medium heat.
- For the vegetables slice the fennel and trim the base of the asparagus
- Using a hot pan, fry the fennel and tomatoes, season with a pinch of black pepper and sea salt.
- Add the asparagus and roast for 10 min at 180°C.
- To serve put the vegetables on a plate and place the pork over, finish with some chopped parsley or chive if wanted.
- For extra flavour reduce the stock to a gravy and drizzle.

- 1 kg pork leg joint
- 2 ltr pork or vegetable stock
- 1 bulb garlic
- 1 tsp black pepper corns
- 4 bay leaves
- 2 whole fennel
- 12 asparagus
- 4 small bunch vine on cherry plum tomatoes
- 1 tsp olive oil
- Sage
- Cracked black pepper
- Pinch sea salt

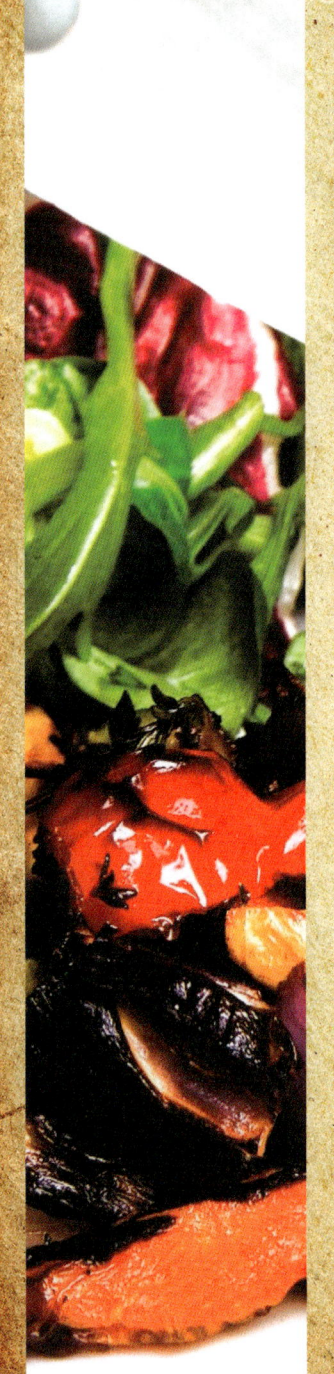

Vegetarian

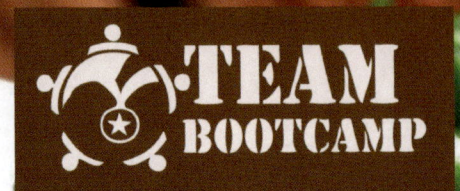

TEAM BOOTCAMP

Ratatouille stuffed aubergine, topped with toasted almonds

Serves - 4

Cooking time – 25 mins

Prep time – 25 mins

INGREDIENTS:

- Slice 2 of the aubergines length ways and hollow out with a spoon leaving 1cm of flesh inside.
- Finely dice the other aubergine along with the courgette, red pepper, tomatoes and onion and chop the garlic and basil.
- Using a hot pan, sweat the onions. Add the red pepper, courgettes and garlic after 2 mins and sweat for a further 5 mins.
- Add the aubergine and tomato and cook for a further 2 mins
- Add the thyme, basil, tomato puree and ho0ney with a pinch of salt and stir thoroughly.
- Remove from the heat and spoon the filling evenly into thyme 4 aubergine halves. Top with almond flakes.
- Cook for 12-15 mins in an oven at 190°C and serve.

- 1 red onion
- 3 aubergines
- 1 red pepper
- 2 beef tomatoes
- 2 sprigs of thyme
- Small bunch of basil
- 2 cloves of garlic
- 1 tbsp. tomato puree
- 20g honey
- 100g almond flakes
- ½ tsp cracked black pepper
- Pinch of sea salt

95

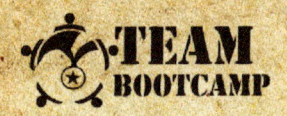

Butternut and almond nut roast

Serves - 6

Cooking time – 30 mins

Prep time – 25 mins

INGREDIENTS:

- Peel, deseed and finely chop the butternut squash.
- Finely chop the onion, carrot, garlic and finely slice and wash the leek.
- Chop the parsley and strip the leaves from the thyme stalks.
- Using a hot pan, sweat the onion, carrots, garlic, leek and squash for 10 min and place in a mixing bowl to cool for 10 mins.
- Add the almonds, egg, thyme, parsley, cumin, celery salt, pepper and a pinch of salt and mix.
- Place on a sheet of cling film and roll out in the cling film to a thick sausage shape.
- Using a Bain Marie, put in the oven, covered in foil at 180°c for 25 mins.
- Remove from the cling film, slice and serve. Can also be served as a larger meal with roast vegetables.

- 1 butternut squash
- 1 red onion
- 1 carrot
- 1 clove of garlic
- 1 leek 200g ground almonds
- 1 egg
- 3 sprigs of thyme
- Small bunch of parsley
- ½ tsp cumin
- ½ tsp celery salt
- ½ tsp cracked black pepper
- Pinch of sea salt

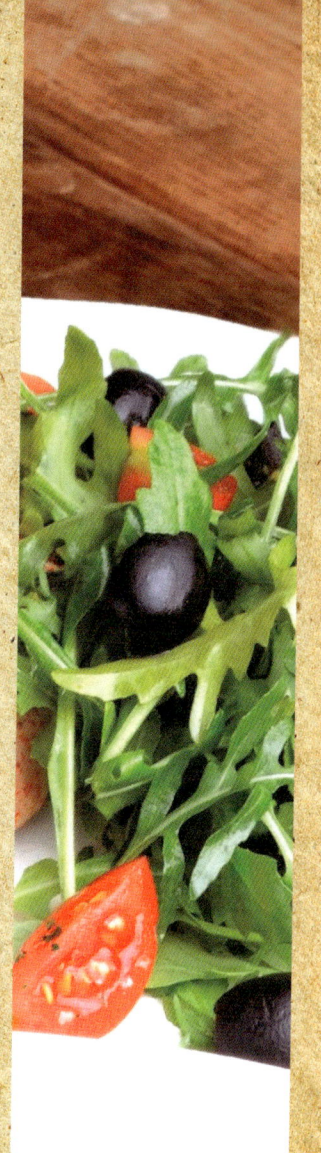

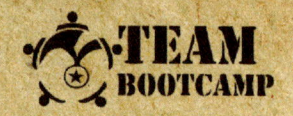

Stuffed sweet potato with spinach, tomato and a macadamia crust

Serves - 4

Cooking time – 20 mins

Prep time – 60 mins

INGREDIENTS:

- Bake the sweet potatoes for 40 mins.
- Finely chop the tomatoes, garlic, onion and chives.
- Using a hot pan, heat the oil and sweat the onion and garlic.
- Add the tomato and chives for 2-3 mins and then remove from the heat.
- Half the sweet potato length ways and hollow out the inside.
- Place sweet potato in a bowl and add the onion, garlic, chives and tomato mix. Finally chop the spinach and add to the mix.
- Mix thoroughly and season with salt and pepper.
- Spoon the mix back into the potato skins and top with chopped macadamia nuts.
- Bake at 190°C for 10 mins and serve.

- 1 tsp olive oil
- 2 large sweet potatoes
- 80g spinach
- 4 tomato's
- 1 clove of garlic
- Small bunch of chives
- 1 onion
- 100g macadamia nuts
- ½ tsp cracked black pepper
- Pinch of sea salt

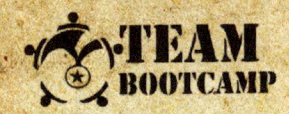

Root vegetable and rosemary stew

Serves - 6
Cooking time – 45 mins
Prep time – 45 mins

INGREDIENTS:

- 4 carrots
- 2 parsnips
- 3 onions
- 2 sweet potato
- 2 leeks
- 500g chestnut mushrooms
- 1 clove of garlic
- Small bunch of rosemary
- 2 tbsp. olive oil
- 125g of Arrowroot
- 1 egg
- 1 litre vegetable stock
- ½ teaspoon cracked black pepper
- Pinch of sea salt

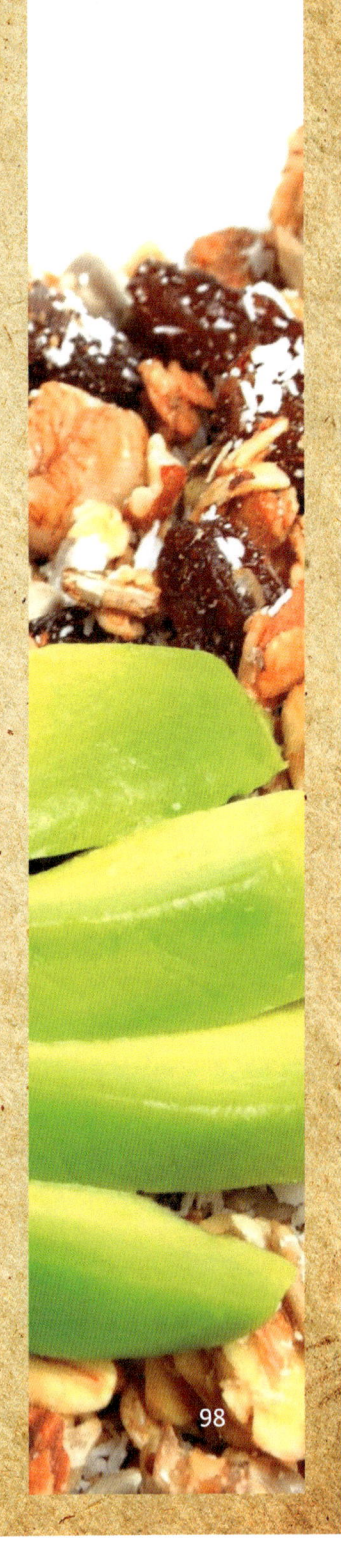

- Wash the veg and chop the carrots, sweet potato, parsnips and onion into 1cm cubes
- Slice the leeks into 1cm think pieces and wash.
- Finely chop the garlic
- Using a hot pan, sweat the onions and garlic in 1 tbsp. of oil for 5 mins then add the carrots, parsnips, potato and leek. Cook for a further 5 mins stirring regularly.
- Add the stock and a few sprigs of rosemary, bring to the boil and then simmer for 35 mins.
- For the dumplings
- Finely chop the mushroom, place on a tray and roast in the oven for 10 mins with a few sprigs of rosemary.
- Place the mushrooms in a bowl and add the arrow root, the last of the oil, 1 egg and salt and pepper. Mix thoroughly and form into 6 even sized balls.
- Place the balls on top of the stew for the last 10 mins of cooking and cover.
- To serve remove the dumplings, season the stew well and scoop into bowls with a dumpling placed on top.

Aubergine and mixed pepper gratin

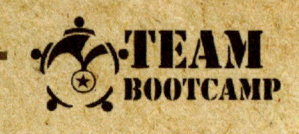

Serves - 4

Cooking time - 35 mins

Prep time - 20 mins

INGREDIENTS:

- Slice the aubergine into 4mm thick discs
- Slice the peppers and onion into large pieces and thinly slice the tomato's.
- Finely chop the garlic.
- In a hot pan, sweat the garlic in a little oil.
- Add the tomato puree, stock and a few sprigs of thyme and simmer.
- In an oven tray, put the peppers, onion and aubergine and roast for 15 mins at 160°C.
- Remove from the tray and put in an oven proof dish.
- Pour over the sauce and top with sliced tomatoes.
- Crumble the feta on top and bake at 160°C for 25 mins.
- Finish with cracked black pepper and serve.

- 1 tsp olive oil
- 2 aubergines
- 1 red pepper
- 1 yellow pepper
- 1 green pepper
- 1 onion
- 2 plum tomato's
- 1 tbsp. tomato puree
- 200 ml vegetable stock
- 1 clove of garlic
- Small bunch of thyme
- 150g of feta cheese
- ½ tsp cracked black pepper
- Pinch of sea salt

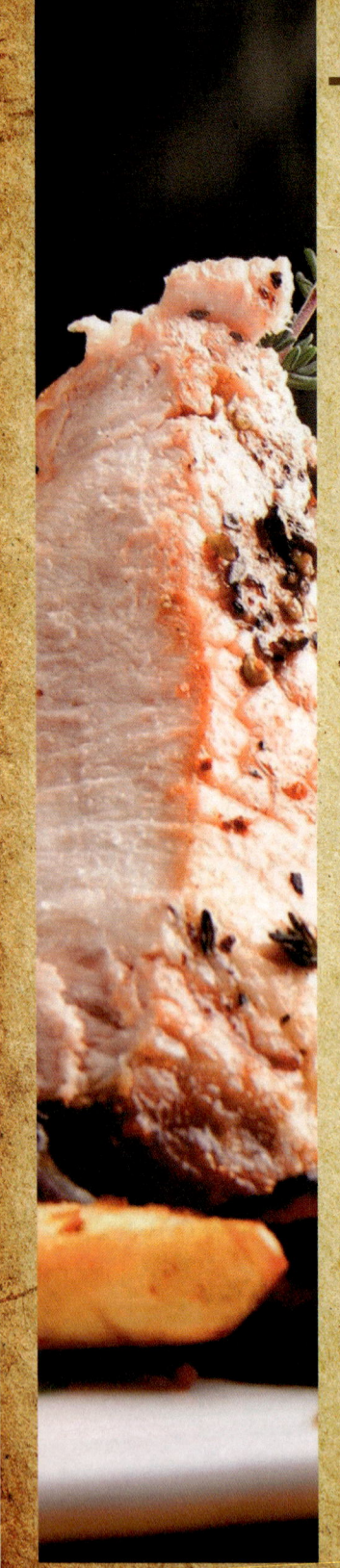

TEAM BOOTCAMP

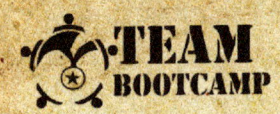

Layered aubergine with courgette, shallot, rocket & basil

Serves - 4

Cooking time – 25 mins

Prep time – 30 mins

INGREDIENTS:

- Slice the aubergine and courgette 4-5mm thick.
- Peel and slice the shallots and garlic.
- Dry roast the aubergine and courgette in the oven at 180°C for 10 mins and then allow to cool.
- Heat the oil in a pan and sweat the shallots and garlic.
- Add the tomato puree, thyme, honey, passatta along with the salt and pepper.
- Shred the basil and rocket and add to the pan.
- In an oven proof dish, place a layer the aubergine and courgette followed by a layer of shallot mix and repeat until all the ingredients have been use, ensuring you finish with a layer of shallot mix.
- Place in the oven at 200°C for 10 mins. Garnish with a little rocket or basil and serve.

- 1 tsp olive oil
- 2 aubergines
- 2 courgettes
- 6 large shallots
- 60g rocket
- 8 basil leaves
- 1 tbsp. tomato puree
- 2 sprigs of thyme
- Cracked black pepper
- 250ml passatta
- 20g honey
- Pinch of sea salt
- 1 clove of garlic

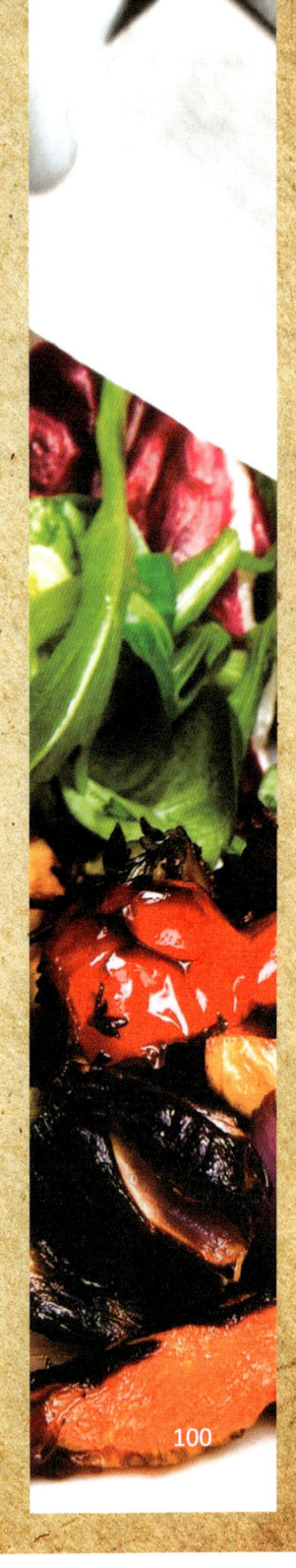

NEW FOR 2015

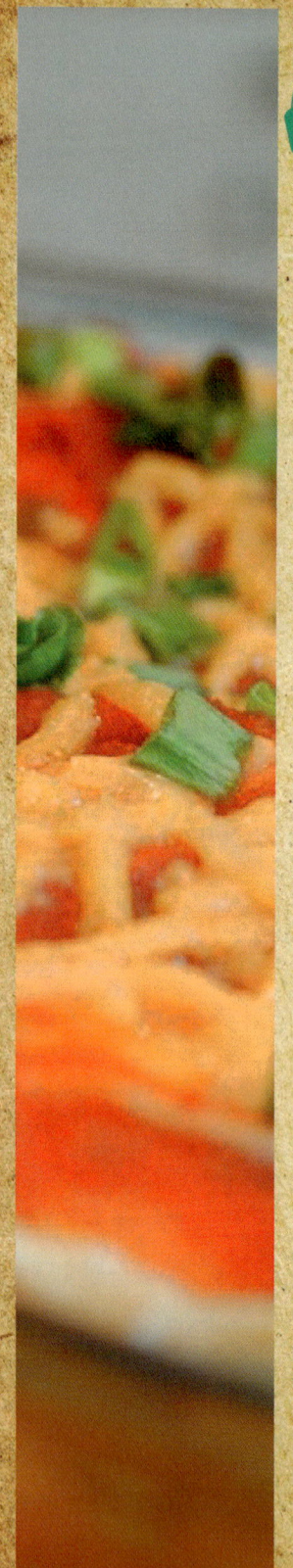

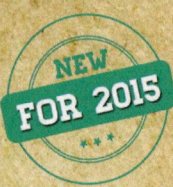

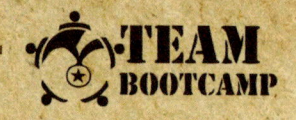

TEAM BOOTCAMP

Spiced Sweet Potato, Spinach & Cashew Casserole

Serves - 6

Cooking time – 65 mins

Prep time – 25 mins

INGREDIENTS:

- Peel and dice both the sweet potato and onion and finely chop the garlic
- Heat the olive oil in a large pan then sweat off the onions for 10 mins before adding the sweet potato and garlic. Cook for a further 10 - 12 mins stirring occasionally and adding the spices after 5 mins and the tomato puree after a further 5 mins and cook for another 2 mins.
- Add stock and garlic and season with black pepper.
- Transfer the mixture into an oven proof casserole dish, sprinkle with the cashews, cover and place in a pre heated oven at 160°c for 60 mins.
- Serve garnished with coriander.

- 1 tbsp tomato puree
- 60g Cashew nuts
- 1 large onion
- 100g Spinach
- 2 cloves of garlic
- small bunch of coriander
- 1 tbsp garam masala
- 1 tbsp turmeric
- 1 tbsp cumin
- 1 tbsp paprika
- 400ml vegetable stock
- Pinch of cracked black pepper
- 1 tsp Olive oil

TEAM BOOTCAMP

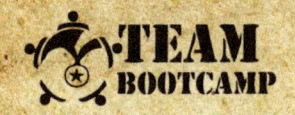

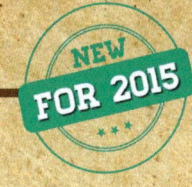

NEW FOR 2015

Vegetable Lasagne

Serves - 4

Cooking time – 60 mins

Prep time – 20 mins

INGREDIENTS:

- Finely dice the carrot, onion and garlic.
- Dice the courgette and tomatoes.
- To act as the 'lasagne sheets - top, tail, peel and deseed the squash and thinly slices length ways.
- Shred the basil and spinach.
- Sweat the onions and carrots in a hot pan for 5 mins then add the garlic and chopped tomatoes. Cook for a further 5 mins.
- Add the courgettes, tomato puree, stock and a pinch of black pepper and simmer for 5 mins then stir in the basil and spinach.
- In an large oven proof dish, layer the sauce with squash with at least 3 layers.
- Crumble feta on top and bake at 160°c for approx. 50 mins until the squash is soft when stabbed with a knife.

- 1 Butternut squash
- 1 Courgette
- 1 Onion
- 3 Plum tomatoes
- 1 Carrot
- 1 tbsp tomato puree
- 2 Cloves garlic
- 200ml vegetable stock
- Small bunch of basil
- 20g feta cheese
- 50g Spinach
- 1 tsp Olive oil
- Cracked black pepper

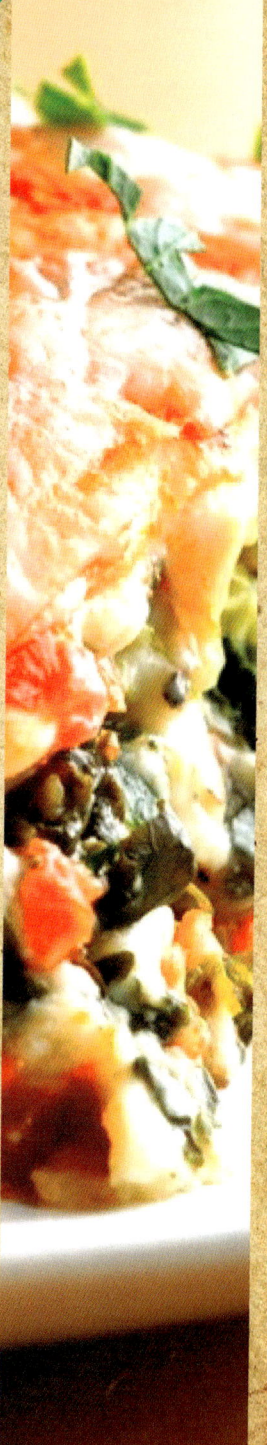

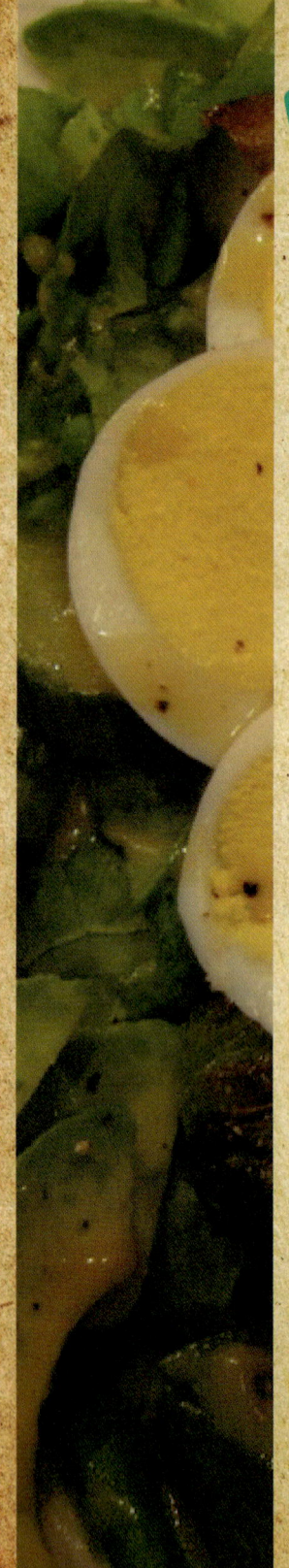

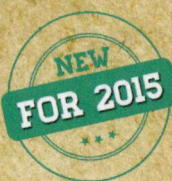

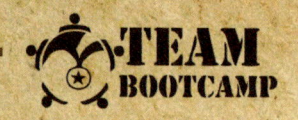

Egg, Asparagus and Avocado Salad

Serves – 4

Cooking time – 20 mins

Prep time – 10 mins

INGREDIENTS:

- Hard boil, cool and peel the eggs and cut into quarters.
- Blanch the asparagus for 90 seconds in boiling water then refresh in cold water until completely cooled.
- With the flesh from avocado dice into small pieces.
- Quarter the tomatoes, peel and slice the onion.
- Put the water cress, rocket, tomatoes, onion and asparagus in a bowl and toss together with olive oil.
- To Serve – Place a hand full of salad mix on the plate then place place 4 quarters of the egg on top and sprinkle with avocado and a pinch of cracked black pepper.

- 4 Eggs
- 12 Asparagus spears
- 2 Avocados
- 50g Water cress
- 50g Rocket
- 4 Salad tomatoes
- 1 Red onion
- 1 tbsp extra virgin olive oil
- Pinch of cracked black pepper

Soups

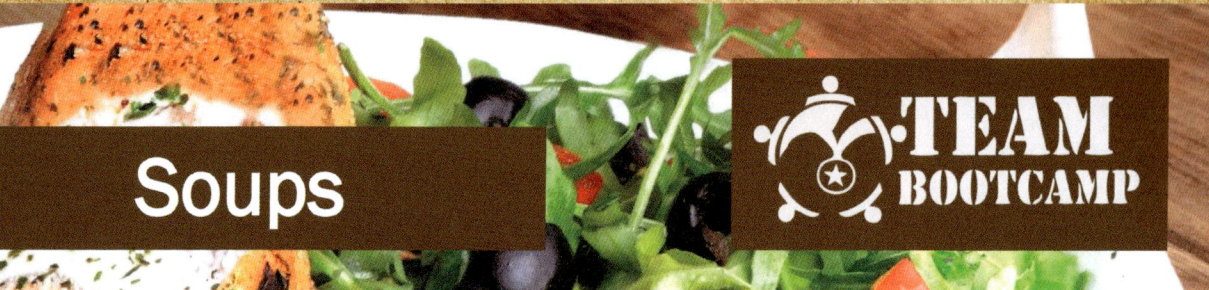

Tomato & Basil

Serves - 6

Cooking time – 45 mins

Prep time - 20 mins

INGREDIENTS:

- Roughly chop onion, celery, carrots, garlic and tomatoes.
- Heat a large pan and sweat the onion, celery, carrots and garlic.
- Add the roughly chopped tomatoes and tomato puree stirring continuously.
- Add honey, passatta and stock and summer for 25 min.
- Blend mix until smooth.
- Pass through a sieve.
- Finely chop basil and add to soup.
- Add pepper to taste before serving.

- 1 large onion
- 2 sticks celery
- 3 clove garlic
- 2 carrots
- 200 g tomato puree
- 10 tomatoes
- 500 ml vegetable stock
- 1 bunch basil
- 1 tsp cracked black pepper
- 30 g honey

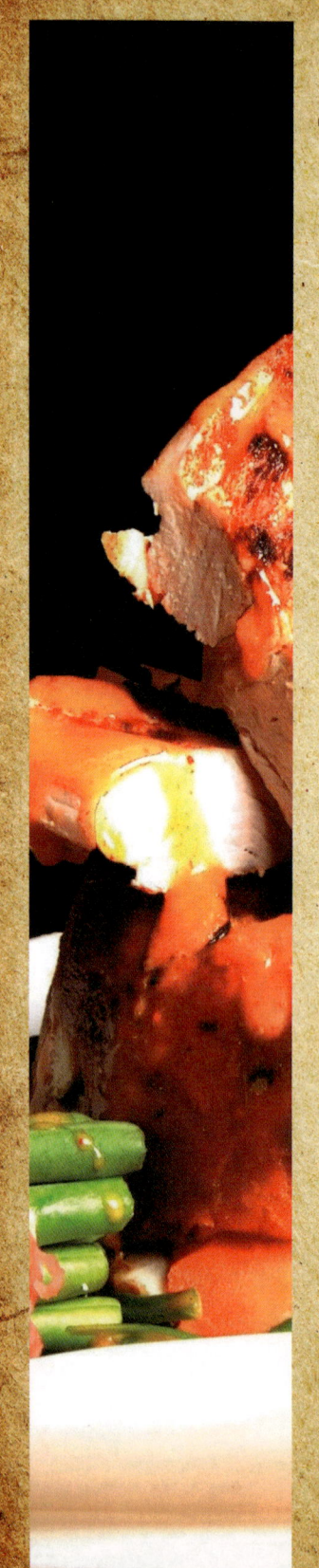

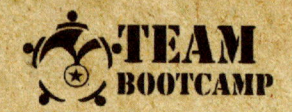

Spiced Butternut Squash & Spinach

Serves - 6

Cooking time – 60 mins

Prep time – 30 mins

INGREDIENTS:

- Peel, de-seed and roughly chop butternut squash.
- Roughly chop onion, garlic and celery.
- Heat up a large pan and add onions, garlic, celery and butternut squash and sweat off for 5 min.
- Add nutmeg and cumin and stir for 2 min.
- Add stock and simmer for 40 min.
- Add spinach and take off the heat and leave for 5 min.
- Blend soup until smooth, it won't need sieved.
- Season with salt and pepper to taste and serve.

- 2 butternut squash
- 1 large onion
- 2 cloves garlic
- 600 ml vegetable stock
- 60 g spinach
- 1/2 tsp nutmeg
- 1 tsp cumin
- 2 stick celery
- Pinch sea salt and cracked black pepper

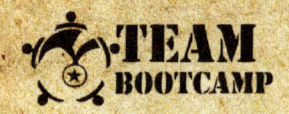

Chicken, Leek & Watercress

Serves - 6

Cooking time – 60 mins

Prep time – 30 mins

INGREDIENTS:

- 2 chicken breasts
- 2 leeks
- 50 g watercress
- 2 onion
- 1 clove garlic
- 1 ltr chicken stock
- 1/2 tsp cracked black
- Small bunch thyme
- Pinch sea salt

- Place chicken breasts in a ovenproof dish and pour 200 mL of stock over them and place into an oven at 190 ºC for 25 min. When done, allow to cool.
- Finely chop the chicken and leeks and place to one side.
- Roughly chop the onion and garlic.
- Using a large pan on a medium heat sweat off the onions and garlic.
- Add 2 sprigs of thyme and stock, simmer for 30 min.
- Take off the heat and blend until smooth.
- Pass the min through a sieve.
- Add the watercress and blend again.
- Add the black pepper and chicken and return to heat for 5 more min.
- Wash the leeks and drain.
- Pan fry the leeks until crispy but not dark in colour.
- Season the soup to taste.
- When serving top the soup with the crispy leeks as a garnish.

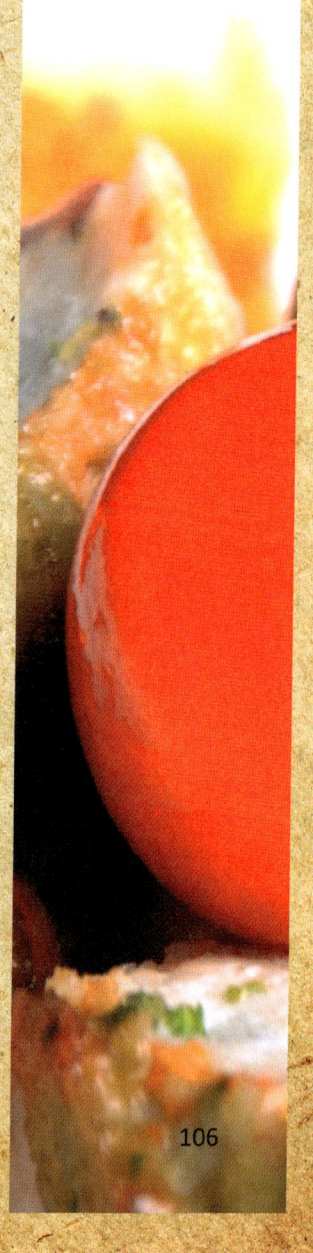

Lamb & Vegetable

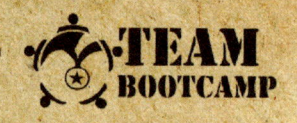

Serves - 6

Cooking time – 90 mins

Prep time – 30 mins

INGREDIENTS:

- Finely dice the lamb, onion, celery, carrots, swede, leeks, butternut squash and garlic
- In a hot large pan brown off the lamb.
- Add the onion, celery, carrot, swede, leeks, butternut squash and garlic and continue to stir for 5 more min.
- Add the stock and rosemary and simmer for 60-80 min.
- Remove the rosemary stalks.
- Add black pepper and remove from heat.
- Season with sea salt to taste before serving.

- 300 g lamb leg
- 1 onion
- 1 stick celery
- 2 carrots
- 1/2 swede
- 1 butternut squash
- 2 leeks
- 1 ltr vegetable or lamb stock
- 1 clove garlic
- Small bunch rosemary
- 1/2 tsp cracked black pepper
- Pinch sea salt

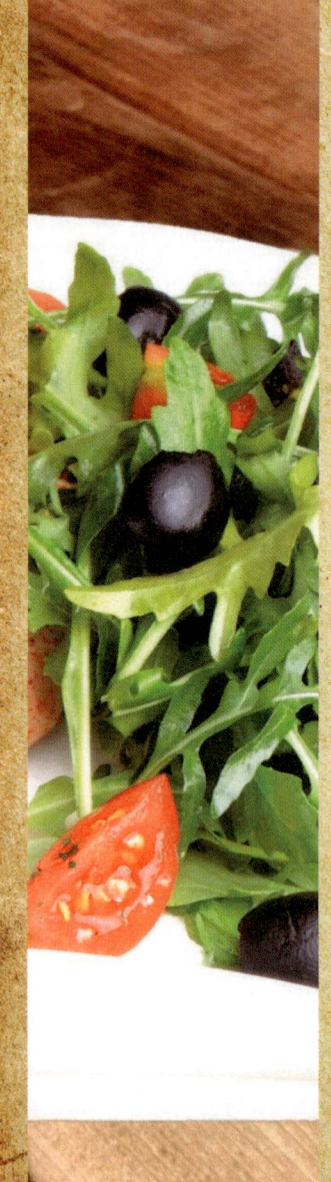

TEAM BOOTCAMP

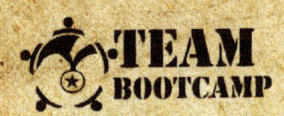

Carrot & Coriander

Serves - 6

Cooking time – 60 mins

Prep time – 35 mins

INGREDIENTS:

- 800 g carrots
- 2 onions
- 1 stick celery
- 900 ml vegetable stock
- 1 bunch coriander
- 1/2 tsp cracked black pepper
- Pinch sea salt
- 1 tsp extra virgin olive oil

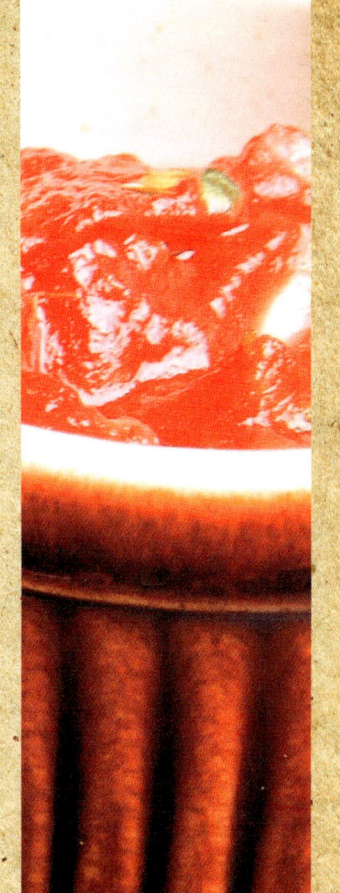

- Roughly chop carrots, celery, onions and garlic.
- In a large hot pot sweat off carrots, celery, onions and garlic in the olive oil.
- Add the stock and allow to simmer for 45 min.
- Blend soup until smooth.
- Pass the soup through a strainer.
- Add the coriander and blend again and add the black pepper.
- Allow to simmer for 5 min and season with sea salt to taste before serving.

NEW FOR 2015

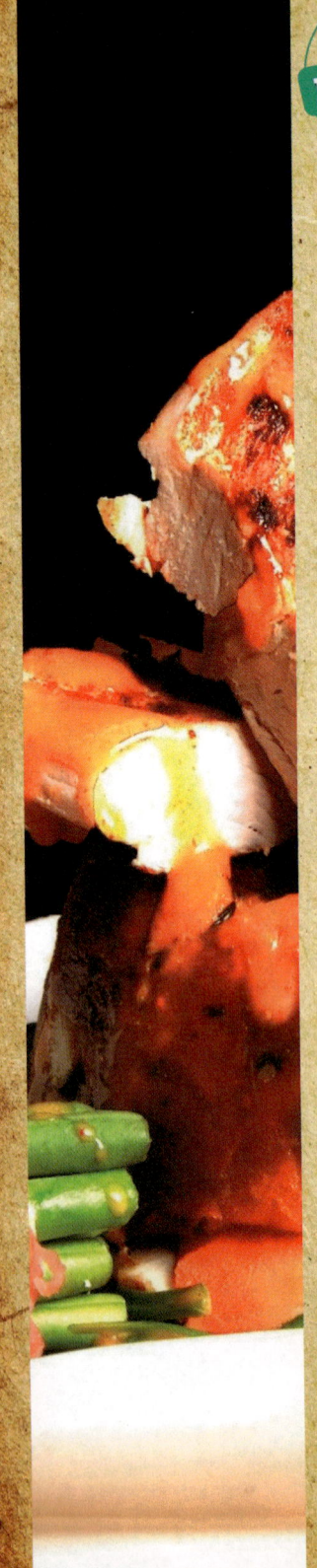

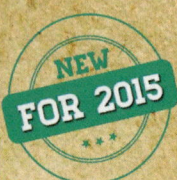

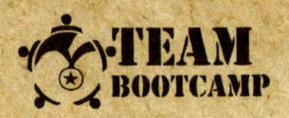

TEAM BOOTCAMP

Beef and tomato soup

Serves - 8

Cooking time – 70 mins

Prep time – 20 mins

INGREDIENTS:

- Heat the oil in a large pan and add the beef and stir until brown.
- Roughly chop the onion, carrot, tomatoes and garlic, add to the beef and continue to cook while stirring for 10-15 mins.
- Add the tomatoes and tomato puree to the mix and stir.
- Add the stock and simmer for 60 mins.
- Once the beef is soft use a blender to blend the soup until thick and smooth.
- Season with pepper and finish with shredded basil to serve.

- 125g diced beef or mince beef
- 100g tomato puree
- 4 plum tomatoes
- 1 onion
- 1 clove of garlic
- 1 carrot
- 800ml beef stock
- Small bunch of basil
- Pinch of cracked black pepper
- 1 tsp of olive oil

Sauce

Stock/Gravy 6 portions

Prep time – 10 mins

Cooking time – 2 hrs.

- Roast off any bones or off cuts of meat until dark in colour
- Roughly chop the carrot, leek, onions and then wash the leeks
- In a large pan brown off the vegetables
- Add the browned bones/meat, garlic and thyme
- After 1 hour add tomato puree
- After 2 hours strain the stock and it's ready to use

INGREDIENTS:

- 300 g carrots
- 1 bulb garlic
- 1 large leek
- 2 onions
- 300-400 g meat off cuts or bones
- 1 tsp tomato puree
- 2 sprigs thyme

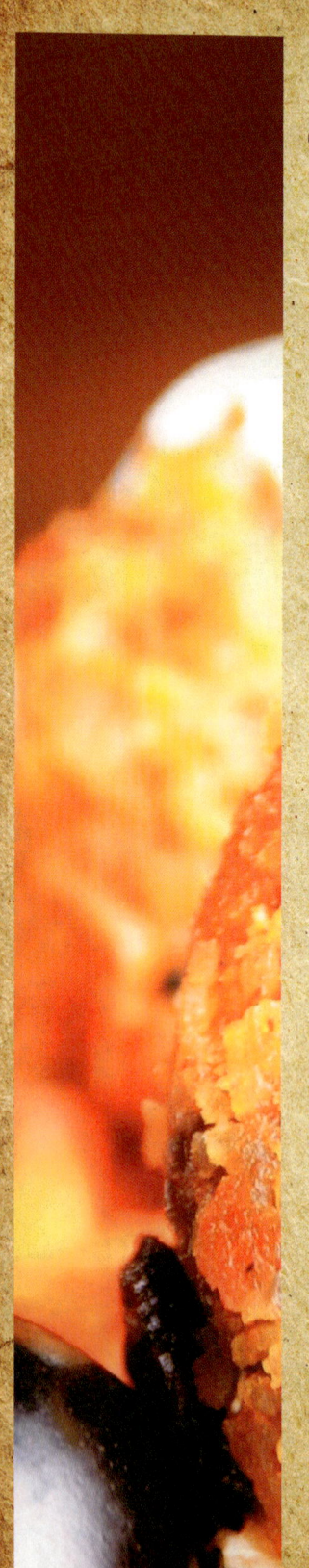

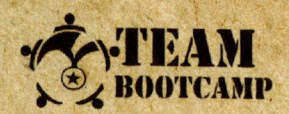

Sweet and Sour Sauce - 6 portions

Prep time – 15 mins   Cooking time – 25 mins

- Finely chop the garlic
- Sweat in a pan gently you don't want to colour it
- Add the vinegar and reduce for 5 mins on a low heat
- Add the honey, tomato puree, stock, fennel seeds, cinnamon, star anise and simmer for 5-10 mins
- In a separate jug add the arrowroot with 1 tsp water and stir till dissolved
- Slowly add the arrowroot mix to the sauce whisking continuously
- Allow to simmer for 5 more mins
- Add black pepper to taste then serve

INGREDIENTS:

- 100 g honey
- 100 g tomato puree
- 50 ml white wine vinegar
- 50 ml fresh chicken or vegetable stock
- 1/4 tsp ground black pepper
- 1/4 tsp fennel seeds
- 1/8 tsp cinnamon
- 1 star anise
- 1 clove garlic
- 1 tbsp arrowroot

Team Bootcamp

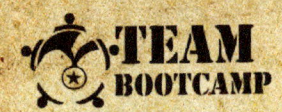

Tomato Ketchup

Prep time – 15 mins **Cooking time – 90 mins**

- Chop the onions and tomatos 1 cm thick
- Sweat of in a large pan
- Add tomato purée, passatta, cloves, celery salt, Worchester sauce, honey and black pepper
- Simmer for 90 minutes
- Blend until smooth
- Pass through a sieve and allow to cool overnight before serving

INGREDIENTS:

- 10 tomatos
- 200 g tomato purée
- 400 ml passatta
- 2 cloves
- 1 onion
- 1/2 teaspoons celery salt
- 1/4 teaspoon Worchester sauce
- 1/2 ground black pepper
- 200 g honey

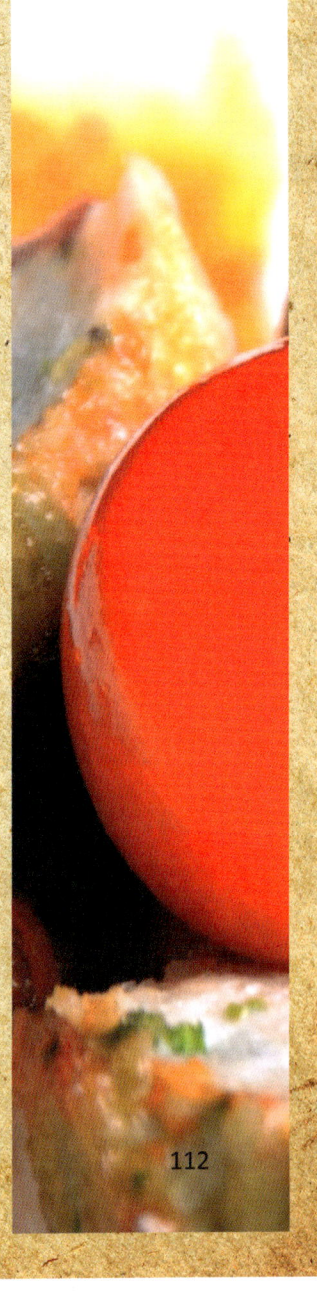

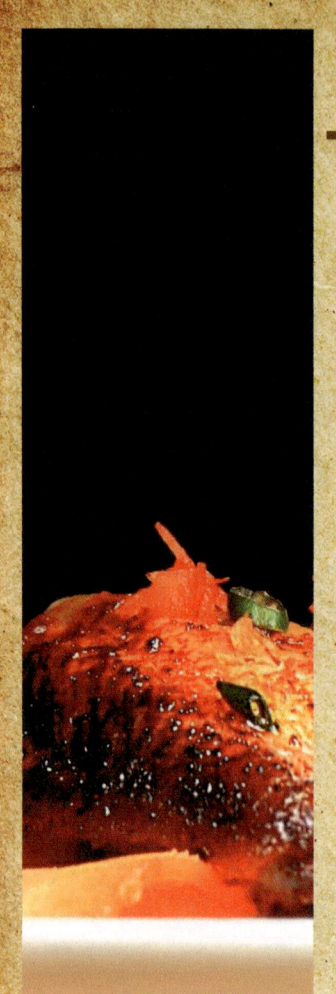

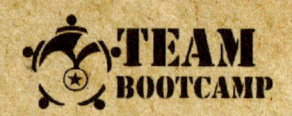

BBQ Sauce

Prep time – 25 mins

Cooking time – 90 mins

- Roughly chop the tomatoes, onion and garlic
- In a hot pan brown onions then add garlic and tomatoes
- Add the vinegar, tomato purée, cloves, celery salt, passatta, Worchester sauce, mustard, honey and bay leaves
- Allow to simmer for 90 mins
- Remove bay leaves and cloves
- Blend until smooth
- Pass through a sieve
- Allowed to rest overnight before serving

INGREDIENTS:

- 60 ml white wine vinegar
- 10 tomatoes
- 200 g tomato purée
- 1 onion
- 2 cloves garlic
- 2 cloves
- 1/2 teaspoon celery salt
- 3 tablespoons Worchester sauce
- 400 ml passatta
- 1 teaspoon mustard (English)
- 1/2 teaspoon black pepper
- 200 g honey
- 2 bay leaves

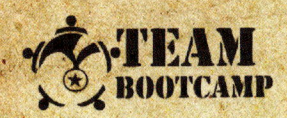

Dairy Free Hollandaise 6 portions

Prep time – 10 mins **Cooking time – 10 mins**

- Separate the eggs as the whites are not needed
- Put the yolks, vinegar, lemon juice and bay leaf in a metal bowl on a Bain Marie and whisk continuously for 30-60 seconds
- Slowly drizzle the oil into the mix while whisking
- When at a nice consistency remove bay leaves
- The sauce should be thick enough to coat the back of a spoon and it's ready to serve

INGREDIENTS:

- 4 egg yolks
- 1 teaspoon white wine vinegar
- 1 teaspoon lemon juice
- 100 ml extra-virgin olive oil
- 1 bay leaf

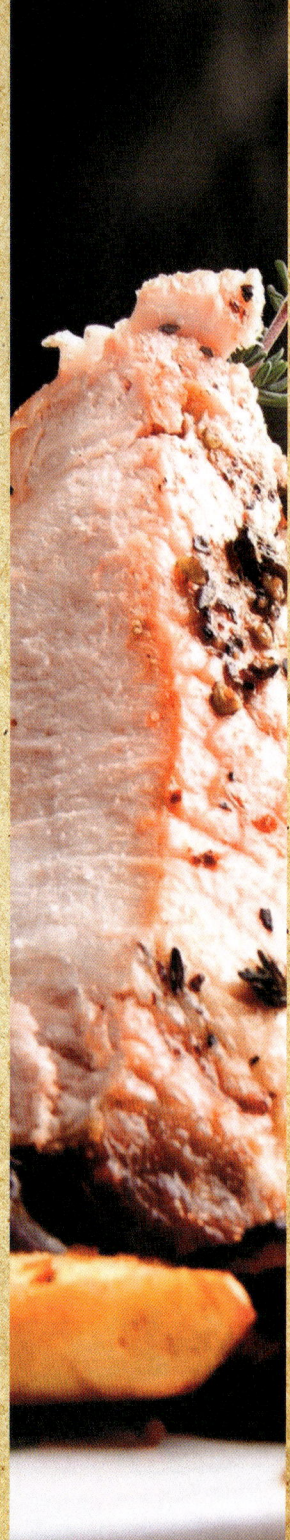

Printed in Great Britain
by Amazon.co.uk, Ltd.,
Marston Gate.